Intermittent Fasting For Women Over 50

The easy way to lose weight, boost your energy and break the spell of aging

By

Evelyn Spring

Respective authors own all copyrights not held by the publisher.

The information herein is offered for informational purposes solely and is universal as so. The presentation of the information is without contract or any type of guarantee assurance.

The trademarks that are used are without any consent, and the publication of the trademark is without permission or backing by the trademark owner. All trademarks and brands within this book are for clarifying purposes only and are the owned by the owners themselves, not affiliated with this document.

Table of Contents

Introduction

You acquire knowledge, strength, and experience as you become older. You form significant bonds with the people around you and watch them blossom. You start to figure out what matters most to you and get rid of many of the restrictions that dominated your childhood. But, in addition to those intangible aspects, your body undergoes changes. Many of these changes that occur with aging are likely familiar to you. For example, your metabolism gradually slows down, making you more prone to heart disease and high blood pressure. You already know not to eat too much salt, and you're probably thinking about restricting items that might raise your cholesterol. Every woman ages differently, yet there are biological factors that contribute to changes like wrinkles and greying hair. Other changes, such as those occurring at the molecular level or in your brain, are absolutely undetectable. As you approach the 2nd half of the century, you will most likely notice a shift in your feelings.

Age-related diseases are ailments and illnesses that become more common as individuals become older, implying that age is a major risk factor. Staying intellectually and physically active may help you look and feel younger, especially if you're in your 50s and starting to notice slight changes in your metabolism or complexion. Many women gain weight during menopause, especially around the belly. Declining estrogen levels, age-related loss of muscular tissue, and lifestyle variables such as food and lack of exercise all contribute to weight increase during menopause.

Women over 50 may benefit from intermittent fasting to lose weight and reduce their risk of acquiring age-related disorders. Intermittent fasting may really reduce blood pressure. Many women above 50 are concerned about reducing weight in addition to seeking to better their health. Lower metabolism, diminished muscle mass, achy joints, and even sleep troubles all make it more difficult to lose weight beyond 50. Simultaneously, declining fat, particularly dangerous belly fat, may significantly lessens your chance of major health problems, which includes heart attacks, diabetes, and cancer. When it refers to weight reduction and minimizing the risk of getting age-related disorders, IF for women over the age of 50 might be a genuine fountain of youth in certain circumstances.

Chapter 1: Women's Body Over 50

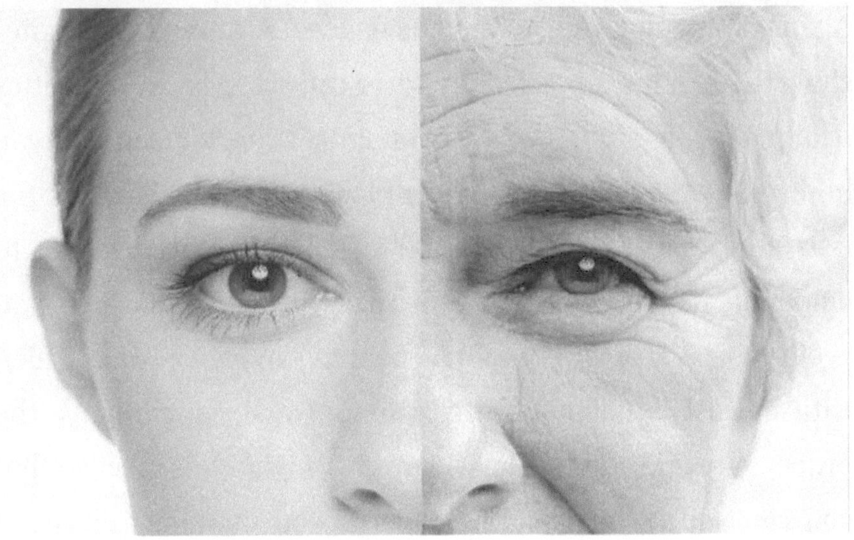

Everyone ages uniquely, and lifestyle factors play a big part, but you'll notice both subtle and obvious changes in your mental and physical health. A lengthy life is a gift that not everyone is fortunate enough to get. However, for those people that do, that blessing is accompanied by certain unavoidable indicators of aging. Your body changes as you grow older, which isn't always a negative thing — it's simply different. Knowing what to anticipate will not only assist you in accepting the changes, but it will also provide you insight into what you could do to make the transition go more smoothly. Some of the changes are subtle and develop over time, while others seem to occur suddenly. It's vital to realize that they're typical, irrespective of when they occur.

1.1 What to Expect at 50?

Age is only a number, as the adage goes. A number of studies show that having a positive mindset can actually lead to better health and longer life. An upbeat mental state, for example, can improve blood sugar levels, lower blood pressure, and lower the risk of heart disease. Even if you're genetically predisposed to dementia, having a good attitude regarding aging may help you avoid it. The answer is to live a healthy, active existence filled with meaningful activities. Of course, you'll want to have the proper screenings as well as be aware of what to expect so that you can address the health concerns you may have ahead of time. It's a wonderful moment in your life to be 50. You accept yourself completely, tell anyone who doesn't like it "stuff you," and try to live a happy and peaceful life. Wouldn't it be wonderful if that were the case all of the time? Unfortunately, it isn't, and although you may have a good life beyond 50, there are several problems that can put a stop to your ambitions or lifestyle. Your body is indeed evolving after 50 years and has a few surprises for you. Let's look at the few most typical shocks in the next years.

1. Food will have a distinct flavor.

Do you recall your Grandma liberally sprinkling salt on your dinner plate? This is due to the fact that your taste receptors are always developing and evolving. The cells that detect aromas diminish in number and are not regenerated as rapidly. But don't simply add salt for flavor; instead, play around with spices to make the meal more interesting.

2. Your sweat would have a distinct odor.

You might have noticed that your smell has altered as you've gotten older. This is due to a reaction by your sweat glands to changes in hormones and, in some situations, drugs.

3. Your cravings will shift.

It's natural to go from sweet towards salty snack desires or vice versa. This is due to shifting and changing hormones, much like your sweat glands. Changes in serotonin levels, for example, have been shown to influence the appetite for sweets, chips, and other goodies.

4. It will be tough to get out of bed in the morning.

Your body is starting to show signs of the previous 50 years' wear and tear; you're not as strong or limber as you once were. In the morning, it's more likely to feel painful and stiff.

5. You'll physically slow down.

Due to the slowing of brain impulses to your muscles, keeping up will become more difficult. Around the age of 40, the brain cells which send motor-control instructions start to decline in most individuals.

6. Dental hygiene needs more attention.

Cavities will resurface, just as they did as a youngster. Tooth enamel deteriorates with time, exposing your teeth to more microorganisms. Brush your teeth two times a day, floss once a day, and visit your dentist on a regular basis to avoid decay.

7. Bruises will become more prevalent.

Because your skin, as you age, becomes thinner and lacks the protection as previously, a little bump might leave a mark.

8. Recovering from an injury may take longer, and you'll have mysterious pains.

Your muscle mass reduces as you age, and your healing systems slow down. Because there is a decline in total strength & a longer healing period, it is essential to keep active and increase strength in order to prevent injury. People in their 50s begin to feel greater physical aches and pains as a result of bad posture or past injuries.

9. Skin will get parched.

Your body starts to create less oil, which really is fantastic for people who suffer from adult acne, but it implies fragile skin for others. To keep skin healthy, remember to use sunscreen and drink plenty of water.

10. You'll probably lose weight.

Due to a decrease in bone density, the spinal column starts to shorten, and menopause implies that new bone cannot be formed as rapidly as it is broken down. Women are more prone to develop osteoporosis as a result of this. Strength training or any activity that exerts stress onto your bones is necessary to inform your brain that new bone cells are being added. It's also critical to consume calcium-rich meals.

11. It's possible that your bladder may become a concern.

An overactive bladder affects a large number of individuals. Because the muscles that regulate the bladder become unstable, contractions occur before the bladder is fully filled. In addition, as you become older, your kidneys produce more pee at night. Constipation

is another issue that often arises. The colon's muscle action slows, changing the mechanics of your body. It's critical to have a high-fiber diet and stay hydrated.

12. Maintaining a healthy weight becomes difficult.

It's increasingly difficult to lose weight & keep it off as your body's metabolisms and hormones alter. To avoid weight gain, make sensible decisions and live a healthy lifestyle.

13. It's impossible to avoid forgetfulness.

Have you realized that you don't remember things as well as you used to? Your brain won't operate as swiftly as it did when you were younger, but you may maintain your mind bright by continuing to engage in highly challenging activities.

14. Sex life will change.

Women may suffer vaginal dryness, and men may notice that sexual erections are much less firm & take longer to raise, but experts advise that taking longer to be completely aroused might help you & your partner become more in sync. Other things that might happen as you become older include:

It's possible that you'll find yourself counting sheep.

People over 50 require the same amount of sleep as younger ones, but they seldom get it. Stress, sadness, and long work hours are common causes of insomnia, but it's also connected to medical disorders, including diabetes, heart disease, and arthritic pain. Weight gain may also cause sleep apnea, a condition in which the body does not obtain enough oxygen, resulting in frequent nighttime awakenings.

Your style may be cramped if your joints are aching:

Osteoarthritis is a condition that affects people over the age of 50 and is caused by wear and strain on the joints as cartilage goes away and bones grind together. Stiffness, Aching, and swelling are all symptoms of the illness.

Weight reduction, which relieves stress onto the joints and strengthens the muscles which support them, is a preventative and also therapeutic lifestyle change. Even if you don't feel like it, avoiding exercising might aggravate arthritis symptoms. In addition, there are over-the-counter and prescription drugs, as well as alternative medical therapies and surgery.

Prepare for a weaker immune system.

Your immune system deteriorates with age, making you more susceptible to illness than you were when you were younger. It's vital to keep your vaccinations up to date. It is critical to maintain a sufficient diet in order to keep our immune systems in fighting form.

You'll have to be extra cautious when it comes to falls.

As you become older, osteoporosis, which is defined by weakening bones that are more prone to shatter, becomes increasingly common. Because of the effects of menopause, the illness is more typically identified in women. Osteoporosis affects around 25% of women over the age of 65 (1 in 4), but it also has impacted about 5% of males over 65 years of age (1 in 20). Weight-bearing workouts promote bone health overall and help avoid osteoporosis-related injuries. Prescription drugs may assist if you've previously been diagnosed with poor bone density. A balanced diet with enough vitamin D & calcium levels, as well as moderate alcohol intake, is also recommended by doctors. It also makes sense to avoid accidents from occurring in the first place by keeping your house secure and clutter-free.

The size of your breasts will change:

After adolescence, a woman's breasts change slowly, while each menstrual month might bring about temporary alterations. The system of the milk duct expands to feed a baby; therefore, the breasts enlarge during pregnancy. As estrogen levels drop after menopause, the breasts alter again, becoming less plump and less elastic, which might cause "sagging." The risk of breast cancer is also increasing: A 30-year-old woman's 10-year risk of acquiring breast cancer is 1 in 227, whereas a 50-year-old woman's 10-year risk is one in 28. Although genetics play a part in breast cancer, you may minimize your risk by keeping a healthy weight, frequently exercising, limiting your alcohol intake, and using hormone replacement treatment for fewer than five years if you need it. All women over the age of 50 should receive a mammogram once a year; if you're between the ages of 50 and 59, or if you're younger, but you have a genetic history of the illness, speak to your doctor regarding whether you should start getting frequent mammography screenings.

You'll notice a decrease in muscle tone and a rise in body fat/weight.

Around the age of 30, your body begins to lose muscle tone and develop fat. As you reach 50, you may have lost a significant amount of muscular mass. According to MedlinePlus, the loss of muscle mass because of aging is only approximately 10% to 15%. The rest stems from a lack of exercise and a bad diet. The great news is that you can preserve or gain muscle tone even if you are beyond 50 years old.

Regular exercise, particularly resistance or strength training, is essential for maintaining and restoring muscle tone. Healthy nutrition goes hand in hand with frequent exercise. These two factors, when combined, may not only improve muscle tone but also reduce body fat. With aging, body fat begins to increase. In this stage of life, a sedentary lifestyle may quickly become ingrained. You feel tired faster than you previously did, so it's easy to get into the routine of doing nothing, particularly nothing physical, on a daily basis. Increased body fat increases your chances of developing illnesses like diabetes. Regular exercise & a nutritious diet may help you maintain a healthy body fat percentage. After age 30, both genders have increases in body fat, but men's weight growth typically stops around 55, while women's weight gain often continues until about 65; from adolescence through menopause, excess weight rest on women's hips & thighs. However, after that, a woman's excess weight is more harmful to belly fat that is linked to an elevated risk of diabetes and heart disease. It's always vital to eat a good diet and exercise to maintain a healthy weight, but it's more critical as you become older.

You'll notice a difference in your hair:

If you're going to grey, it'll most likely begin in your 50s, but some women may start sooner (it's entirely genetic). However, as you get older, your hair thins down and grows slowly. Don't be frightened if you've seen additional strands in your hair brush recently. Almost everyone loses hair over time, particularly beyond the age of 50. Female pattern baldness begins with a broadening of the center hair part that extends to the top and crown of the head. It is a hormone-related disorder that may be inherited. Unlike male baldness, it seldom affects a woman's whole head of hair. You may increase the health of your hair regardless of your age or condition by preventing harsh chemicals & treating it carefully. Remember that when you go through these & other changes, time provides a lot of advantages.

Pelvic & reproductive health would deteriorate.

Strong muscles & ligaments that hold your pelvic floor are essential for your sexual, reproductive, & urinary health. Changes in the body caused by childbirth, hysterectomies, &

menopause may lead to illnesses, including pelvic organ prolapse, which occurs when the pelvic organs fall out of position, and urine incontinence, which is the inability to regulate urination. Preventing these problems may be as simple as keeping pelvic-floor & core strength. Kegels, the most basic exercise for the pelvic floor, is straightforward: Pretend you're keeping in gas for ten seconds with an empty bladder, then relax for ten seconds. 3-5 times a day, do five to ten repetitions. Menopause also results in thinner, drier vaginal tissue, making sex less pleasurable.

1.2 Health Disorders in Women after 50

Cardiovascular Diseases:

In the US, heart diseases are the top cause of death, and it is also among the major reason of death in a number of other nations. Coronary artery disease is the most prevalent kind, which includes a blockage or narrowing of the major arteries providing blood to the heart. Obstructions may form over time or suddenly, as in a rupture, resulting in potentially deadly heart attacks. Heart disease is more likely to develop as you get older, and it is more common in those over the age of 50. Women over the age of 50 are more likely to have cardiac problems such as cerebrovascular disease, high blood pressure, arteriosclerosis, etc.

Cancer

Age is one of the most important risk factors since many forms of cancer develop as you get older, in which aberrant cells develop out of control. As per the American Cancer Society, adults over the age of 55.5, especially women, are diagnosed with 77 percent of all malignancies. Cancer is the biggest cause of mortality in both men & women in Canada. Skin, lung, breast, colorectal, bladder, prostate, non-lymphoma, Hodgkin's & stomach cancers are among the malignancies that become more frequent as you get older.

Type 2 Diabetes

Diabetes is a condition that affects how your body consumes glucose (sugar) from the food you eat. Type 1 diabetes (also known as juvenile diabetes) is a type of diabetes that affects persons under 30 years of age & causes the bodies to cease making insulin. Type 2 diabetes, which is significantly more frequent, develops after the age of 50 and includes insulin resistance, causing the body to handle glucose inappropriately. Both kinds of diabetes cause dangerously high blood sugar levels, which may result in heart attacks, strokes, nerve damage, renal failure, and blindness.

According to research by the Centers for Disease Control & Prevention, the occurrence of type two diabetes is already on the rise, yet the rate of development seems to have decreased

(CDC). Adopting healthy behaviors, such as frequent exercise & eating a well-balanced diet, helps maintain levels of blood glucose in a normal range and avoid health decline before or after the beginning of diabetes.

Parkinson's disease

This degenerative neurological illness produces stiffness, tremors, and halting movement and is named after the British physician that initially characterized it in the early 1800s. Though age is just one risk factor, 3/4th of all Parkinson's disease cases begin beyond the age of 50. Parkinson's disease affects women above the age of 50. The disorder is thought to be produced by a mix of genetics and environmental factors, such as exposure to chemicals, according to researchers. Traumatic brain injuries, according to research, may also play a role.

Dementia (Including Alzheimer's disease)

Memory loss, mood swings, confusion, trouble speaking, and poor judgment are all symptoms of dementia, which is caused by a progressive decline in brain function. Alzheimer's disease is one of the most prevalent causes of dementia. However, it may also be caused by a variety of other conditions, including:

- Dementia is linked to vascular disease (due to the impaired blood flow towards the brain)

- Frontotemporal disorders

- Lewy body dementia

- Lewy body dementia

- Parkinson's Disease

While dementia is more common as people become older, it is not a normal part of the aging process.

COPD (Chronic Obstructive Pulmonary Disease)

COPD (Chronic obstructive pulmonary disease) is characterized by a decrease in airflow into & out of the lungs as a result of inflammation in the airways, thickening of the lining of the lungs, and excessive mucus formation in the air tubes. Women People over the age of 5 are more likely to get COPD. It is not possible to cure the disorder, but it could be treated and, perhaps more significantly, avoided. Among the signs and symptoms are:

- A cough that is becoming worse and is persistent

- Wheezing

- Breathing problems

Chronic exposure to airborne irritants such as tobacco smoke (whether as a primary or a second-hand smoker), occupational pollutants, or industrial pollution is the major cause of COPD. The most major risk factor is still cigarette smoking.

Osteoarthritis

Osteoarthritis is the most prevalent type of arthritis and a degenerative joint condition. Osteoarthritis becomes more frequent as individuals become older, and it affects more women than men. You are also more prone if you have genetics, are obese, or have had a previous joint injury. Osteoarthritis is characterized by swelling and discomfort in the joints. It may be treated with anti-inflammatory or pain-relieving drugs, as well as lifestyle changes such as weight reduction, exercise, and physiotherapy.

Osteoporosis

Osteoporosis, sometimes known as the "brittle bone disease," is characterized by a decrease in bone mass, resulting in thinning & weakening bones. It becomes more frequent as women become older, particularly in Caucasian & Asian women and also those from colder climates like Scandinavia, where vitamin D insufficiency is widespread. It's also one of the risk factors if you have osteopenia or poor bone density. According to National Osteoporosis Foundation, up to half of all women over 50, as well as 27% of males over 50, may break a bone as a result of osteoporosis. Hip fracture is a severe concern for elderly people since they cause loss of mobility and, in around one-quarter of all the cases, mortality within one year of injury.

Regular weight-bearing activity, a calcium- and vitamin-D-rich diet, and quitting smoking may all assist in preventing osteoporosis.

Cataracts

A cataract is a cloudiness inside the lens of the eye that develops over time due to a variety of factors, such as aging, smoking, UV light exposure, and diabetes. The National Institutes of Health estimates that half of all persons over 60 years of age have a cataract or have undergone cataract surgery. You might not notice a cataract at first, but vision might become blurry and limited over time. Cataract surgery to remove & replace the lens may be recommended. It may now be done as an outpatient treatment in as little as an hour, thanks to technological developments.

Hearing Loss

Due to the degeneration of microscopic hairs inside your ear that assist process sound, hearing loss is normal as you get older. Simple hearing changes, like difficulty following a discussion in a noisy environment, difficulty identifying specific consonants (particularly at higher voices), some sounds being louder than normal, and voices looking muffled, may all be signs of hearing loss. A number of variables, other than your age, may impact how well you can hear as you become older, including persistent exposure to loud sounds, smoking, and heredity. Age-related hearing loss affects around 25% of those aged 65 to 74 and 50% of those aged 75 and over.

Disorders Related to Menopause:

Menopause starts when menstrual cycle finishes. Menopause isn't a medical illness, and some women see it as a time of empowerment. Hormonal fluctuations and other variables, but at the other hand, might be aggravating. As they approach menopause, many women experience physical symptoms like night sweats, hot flashes, vaginal dryness, and reduced sex desire. Anxiety, mood fluctuations, and a reduction in sex desire are all possible side effects.

These symptoms may occur after or before menstruation and can last for months or years. The quality of a person's life may be influenced in a number of ways. However, there are methods for dealing with these symptoms. Each woman is affected differently by menopause. During and after the shift, many individuals have full, active lives, and others are glad to be free from menstruation & birth control. Eating a balanced diet and exercising on a regular basis may help an individual feel better and enhance their general health in the long term. For those suffering from menopausal symptoms, there are treatments and resources available.

Symptoms:

Various mental and physical changes may occur around menopause, resulting in symptoms. Some of these symptoms occur before and after menopause. The following are some of the changes that occur during peri-menopause and menopause:

Fertility issues:

Estrogen levels begin to diminish when a woman is near the end of her reproductive period but before menopause. This lowers the likelihood of getting pregnant.

Irregular menstruation:

Periods becoming less regular is generally the first symptom that menopause is approaching. They might appear more often or less regularly than normal, and they could be heavier or lower in weight. Anyone who is concerned about their menstrual cycle must see a doctor since these changes might signal pregnancy or other health problems.

Pain and dryness in the vaginal area:

In the vaginal region, there is a lot of dryness and soreness. During peri-menopause, dryness, itching, and pain in the vaginal region may start and remain until menopause. A woman with these signs may experience chafing and pain during vaginal intercourse. Additionally, infection is a hazard if the skin breaks. Atrophic vaginitis, which is characterised by the dryness, weakening, and inflammation of vaginal wall, may develop after menopause. A range of moisturizers, lubricants, and medications may be used to treat vaginal dryness and associated problems.

Hot flashes:

Hot flashes are common throughout the menopausal period. They cause a person to feel a sudden surge of warmth in his or her upper body. The feeling may start in the face towards the neck, or chest and go up or down the body. A heat flash may also cause:

- Sweating causes red patches to form on the skin.

- Some people have nighttime sweats & cold flashes, or chills, in addition to or instead of hot flashes.

Disruptions in sleep:

Sleep issues are common during menopause and may be caused by a variety of factors, including:

- anxiety

- sweating during night

- a greater desire to urinate

Getting lots of exercises & avoiding big meals before night may assist with these problems, but if they don't go away, see a doctor.

Emotional changes:

Depression, anxiety, and poor mood are among symptoms of menopause. It's normal to have bouts of rage and sobs. Hormonal swings and sleep interruptions might worsen these issues. It's also possible that a person's sentiments about menopause have a role. Worries about a lack of libido or the loss of fertility might increase depression throughout menopause. While feelings of sorrow, rage, and weariness are common throughout menopause, they're not invariably signs of depression. Anyone who's been depressed for two weeks or more should seek medical help, as they will be able to recommend the right plan of action.

Having difficulty concentrating and learning:

Two-thirds of women have symptoms in the months leading up to menopause. Women may have trouble concentrating and remembering things. Having a healthy diet, being physically and intellectually engaged, and having an active lifestyle may all assist with these concerns. Finding a new pastime or joining some club or local activity, for example, might be beneficial to certain individuals.

Physical changes

Around the phase of menopause, many bodily changes might occur. A deposit of fat all around the abdomen may occur, as well as a weight increase.

- Hair color, texture, & volume changes

- breast Tenderness & reduction

- urinary incontinence

The relationship between these alterations and menopause, on the other hand, is not always evident. Some may occur simultaneously with the shift, and age & lifestyle may also play a major role.

1.3 Weight Gain

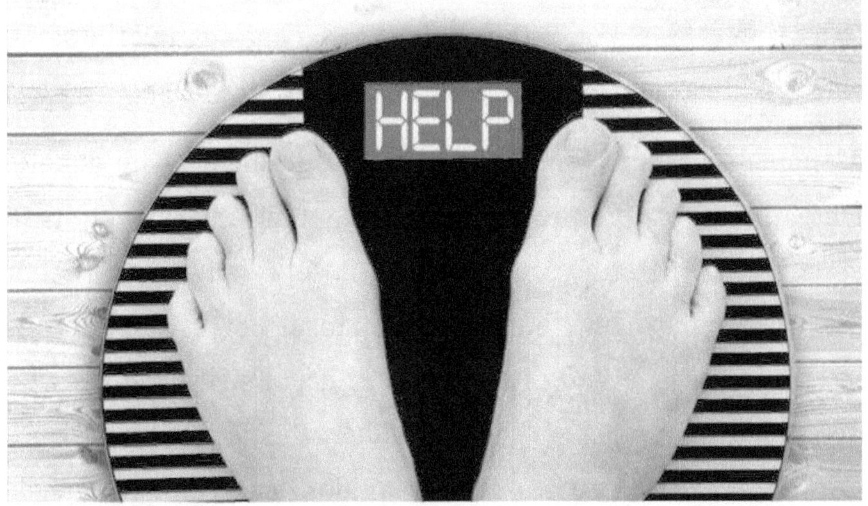

You may realize that maintaining your normal weight gets more challenging as you grow older. In fact, most women gain weight as they approach menopause. However, weight increase after menopause is not unavoidable. You may change your life by focusing on good eating habits and maintaining an active lifestyle.

Causes of weight gain:

Menopause's hormonal changes may cause you to acquire weight around your midsection rather than your thighs and hips. However, hormonal changes alone may not always result in weight increases during menopause. In most cases, the weight increase is caused by age, and also lifestyle and hereditary factors. Muscle mass, for example, declines as people become older, but fat levels rise. The pace at which the body burns calories slows down as you lose muscle mass (metabolism). It may be more difficult to keep a healthy weight as a result of this. You'll gain weight if you keep eating the same way you always do and don't improve your physical activity.

Menopause weight gain might also be influenced by genetic factors. You're more prone to gain weight around the abdomen area if your parents or any other close relatives do. Other factors that may contribute to menopausal weight gain include lack of exercise, a bad diet, and insufficient sleep. People who don't have enough sleep are more likely to snack and eat more calories. Gaining weight may have major health consequences. Excess weight, particularly around the middle, raises your risk of a variety of problems, including:

- Breathing difficulties

- Diseases of the heart and blood vessels

- Diabetes type 2

Excess weight raises your chance of developing malignancies such as breast, colon, and endometrial cancers. Your muscles lose size as you get older, and your metabolism slows down. Weight gain at the time of menopause may be produced by these changes. Other bodily changes that may occur with menopause include:

- Changes in the skin, like dryness and elasticity loss

- Dryness of the vaginal canal

- Hair development (or loss).

These changes may have an impact on a woman's body image and self-esteem and also her risk of sexual problems and depression. Taking action to control menopausal symptoms may assist. Other factors that contribute to weight increase during menopause include:

- Age.

- Muscle mass loss and decreased physical activity

- children's number

- Obesity that runs in the family

- usage of Antidepressant and antipsychotic medicines

- chemotherapy

- metabolic rate slowed

- A different way of life, such as dining out more.

1.4 Managing your Weight

There is no secret method for avoiding or reversing weight gain after menopause. Simply follow these weight-loss guidelines: Increase your physical activity. Physical activity, such as aerobic exercise & strength training, may aid in weight loss and weight maintenance. Your body uses calories more effectively as you grow muscle, making it simpler to maintain a healthy weight. Experts suggest moderate aerobic exercise, like brisk walking, for 150 minutes at least per week for most healthy individuals, or strenuous aerobic activity, like running, for 75 minutes at least per week for most healthy adults.

- Strength training activities should also be done at least 2 times a week. You may need to work out more if you really want to shed weight or reach certain fitness objectives.

- Consume fewer calories. You may require around 200 fewer calories per day in your 50s than you needed in your 30s and 40s to maintain your present weight, much alone remove extra pounds.

- To reduce calories without compromising nutrition, pay very good attention to the things you eat & drink. More vegetables, fruits and whole grains, particularly those foods which are less processed and richer in fibre, should be ingested.

- A plant-based diet is often healthier than other alternatives, according to the finest bariatric surgeon in Nashik. Legumes, almonds, salmon, soy, and low-fat dairy products are also good options. Red meat and poultry, in particular, should be taken in moderation. Stick margarine, Butter, and shortening may all be replaced with oils like olive or vegetable oil.

- Examine your sweet tooth. In the typical American diet, added sugars make up roughly 300 calories per day. Sweetened beverages, like soft drinks, energy drinks, juices, flavored waters, as well as sweetened tea and coffee, account for around half of these calories.

- Cookies, cakes, pies, ice cream, doughnuts, and candy are among the items that lead to excessive dietary sugar.

- Alcohol should be used in moderation. Alcoholic drinks raise the risk of weight gain by adding extra calories to your diet.

- Seek assistance. Surround yourself with friends and family who will encourage your attempts to eat a healthy balanced diet more. Even better, form a group and make the necessary lifestyle adjustments together.

Crash diets should be avoided.

A crash diet entails drastically lowering your food intake in a short period of time. Because of the alterations in your muscles, you are more prone to gaining weight when you resume your usual eating habits. Leptin (sometimes known as the "fat hormone") plays a crucial function in body weight regulation by influencing appetite and metabolic rate. According to studies, when you go on a crash diet, your Leptin levels decrease, which raises your hunger and lowers your metabolism.

Intermittent Fasting:

When it comes to losing weight, women over 50 often have a difficult time. This may be caused by a variety of factors. The most common cause is a slowed metabolism. The quicker your metabolism is, the leaner muscle you will have. However, as you age, you shed lean muscle mass & become less active than you once were. What's the end result? Stubborn body fat, which refuses to go away. Intermittent fasting has grown in popularity in recent years as a result of its many health advantages and the truth that it does not limit your meal choices. Fasting has been shown to boost mental health and metabolism and perhaps prevent various malignancies, according to research. It may also protect women over 50 against a certain nerve, muscle, and joint diseases. In the next chapters of this book, the benefits of intermittent fasting for women over 50 are described in further detail.

Chapter 2: Introduction to Intermittent Fasting and its Benefits

Intermittent fasting (IF) refers to a category of calorie-restricted (CR) diets wherein the dieter switches between times of fasting (typically defined as simply drinking water or no-calorie drinks) and periods of non-fasting. Most weight reduction diets are based on meal plans, recipes, food lists, calorie counting, or other similar characteristics. IF is focused on time intervals rather than meal plans, recipes, food lists, calorie counting, or other similar elements.

2.1 History of Fasting

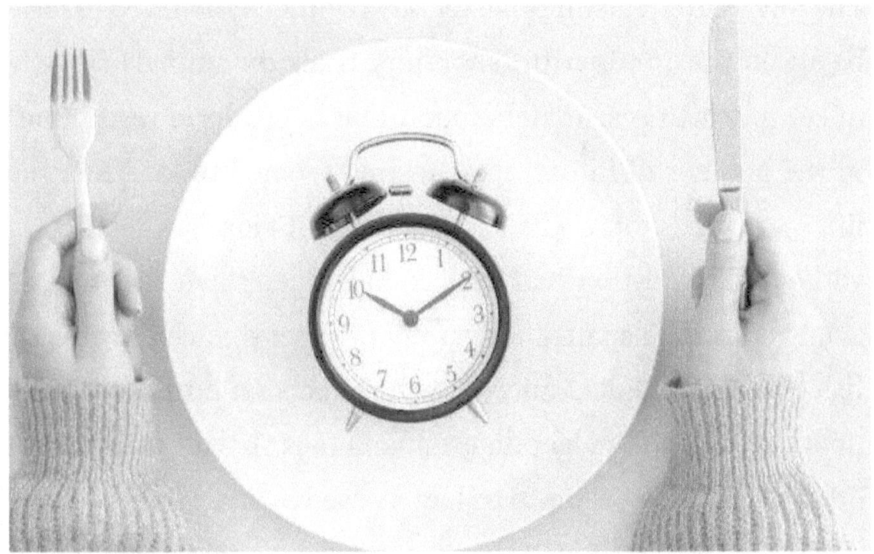

Fasting is not a new notion. Humans have fasted for a variety of reasons, including nighttime periods, religious reasons, and food shortages. Fasting is said to be one of the world's oldest therapeutic practices. Fasting was recommended by Hippocrates of Cos, a Greek scholar. Fasting was also strongly advocated by other Greek scholars like Plato and Aristotle. Fasting was thought to be a universal tendency for a variety of ailments by the ancient Greeks. They also believed that it enhanced cognitive ability. Consider a day when your tummy was overflowing with food. Did you feel cognitively alert and energized afterward, or were you drowsy and sleepy? Fasting is used to wash or purify the soul in several faiths (including Islam, Christianity, and Buddhism). However, it effectively translates into the identical advantages that the Greek researchers have approved.

The intermittent fasting-like dietary regimen is believed to have begun in the 1940s with laboratory trials on animals (mostly mice) in which researchers found that CR (calorie restriction) in the manner of intermittent fasting seemed to lengthen the life spans of the animals. Calorie restriction without malnutrition has been found to lengthen the median & maximum life spans in a variety of species, including yeast, fish, & dogs, and also mice, but the effects on humans are yet unknown due to the fact that human life is shorter than that of other animals. IF seems to be largely used by male bodybuilders and sportsmen in industrialized nations, who might combine it with other sorts of diet cycling regimes. Food cycling is the practice of certain weightlifters of reversing the amounts of fats and carbs in their diet according to the phase of their training schedule, low fat/high carbohydrate usually on training days & high fat/low carbohydrate on rest days.

Modern IF (intermittent fasting) is all about progressively adopting fasting into your daily diet. It entails eating wisely most of the time and then going without food for an extended length of time every now and then. You may also have cheat days once a week when you can overeat a restricted quantity of food.

2.2 How IF Works

You won't have to starve yourself if you practice intermittent fasting, sometimes known as IF. When you don't fast, it also doesn't give you permission to eat a lot of unhealthy stuff. Rather than eating snacks and meals throughout the day, you eat inside a set period of time. The majority of individuals adhere to an IF regimen that demands people to fast for twelve to sixteen hours per day. They consume regular meals and snacks in the remaining time. Because most individuals sleep for roughly eight hours during their fasting hours, sticking to this type of eating window isn't as difficult as it seems. You're also recommended to consume zero-calorie beverages, including tea, water, and coffee. You'll receive the greatest effects from this diet if you stick to it. At the very same time, on exceptional occasions, you may surely take a vacation from this type of eating routine. You should try several types of intermittent fasting to see which one works best for you. Many patients begin their IF journey with the twelve-hour schedule and subsequently advance to the 8-hour plan. After then, attempt to keep to your strategy as closely as possible.

Some individuals claim that IF has helped them lose weight simply because the short eating window forces them to eat fewer calories. For example, instead of three meals and two snacks, they may only have the time for two meals & one snack. They become more conscious of the foods they eat and prefer to avoid processed carbohydrates, bad fats, and empty calories. Of course, you have the freedom to eat any healthful foods you choose. While some individuals use intermittent fasting to lower their total calorie consumption, others use it in conjunction with a vegan, keto, or another diet. It may be surprising that merely changing your eating schedule will promote weight loss. Despite this, your bodies react to fasting in a positive manner. When your body goes into fasting mode, your fat reserves are called upon to be utilized as fuel, leading you to burn fat for energy. Of course, just because you're not fasting doesn't mean you can eat anything you want. To get the greatest outcomes, eat healthy whole foods, unprocessed carbs, and lean meats. Keep in mind that calorie-free beverages such as tea, black coffee, and water may be consumed during fasting times! You may even notice that you are eating more slowly and with more enjoyment.

Increase in Metabolism:

Surprisingly, evidence indicates that IF has the same or less detrimental effects on metabolism as typical diets. Many people believe that intermittent fasting increases metabolism since it results in less lean body mass loss and more fat burning. Although it's hard to reduce weight without losing some lean body mass, evidence shows that intermittent fasting loses a smaller proportion of lean body mass than standard dieting. The body's calorie-burning rate reduces when lean body mass is preserved. Short fasting periods, on the other hand, lead the body to access fat reserves and burn a higher proportion of fat mass to produce energy. Many people think that skipping meals causes your body to adjust by slowing down your metabolism in order to save energy. It's commonly known that going without eating for lengthy periods of time might induce a reduction in metabolism.

Short-term fasting, on the other hand, has been demonstrated to speed up rather than slow down your metabolism. Previous research of 11 healthy men revealed that a three-day fast raised their body metabolism by a whopping 14 percent. This increase is assumed to be linked to an increase in the fat-burning hormone norepinephrine.

Autophagy and IF:

Autophagy is a normal cellular activity that permits your cells to digest unnecessary or damaged components. Autophagy is a biological process that helps the cell function normally (homeostasis). The term "autophagy" literally means "self-eating."

Autophagy looks to be self-destruction, however it really aids in the removal of harmful material and rejuvenation of cells. Autophagy may either completely destroy damaged molecules or recycle them into new parts that can be used for cellular repair. When cells are deprived of nutrients or oxygen, autophagy may offer an alternative energy source from recycled cellular material, allowing them to survive. Autophagy may help the immune system by removing toxins and harmful microorganisms. Under some conditions, autophagy may also result in planned cell death (apoptosis). In a word, autophagy is a cellular mechanism that balances the synthesis and elimination of cellular components to preserve cell homeostasis.

Intermittent fasting may be used to trigger autophagy. Under normal circumstances, when cell has adequate nutrients, autophagy removes damaged parts in the cell. Autophagy aids in the breakdown of a few of the cellular constituents when these cells are deprived for energy, enabling the cells to thrive. Excess glucose gets stored as glycogen in the liver. When glucose levels decline owing to fasting, the liver converts glycogen to glucose & releases it. When the liver's glucose reserves run out, it decomposes fat to make ketones, which provide energy. This state is referred to as ketosis. To reduce weight, many individuals use intermittent fasting & calorie restriction diets. A typical diet called as the keto diet, in which fat contributes for 75% of daily calories, is hypothesized to promote ketosis and autophagy. There aren't enough research on the long-term effects of the ketogenic diet. According to studies, autophagy may be activated by calorie restriction, intermittent fasting, and ketosis.

2.3 IF Methods

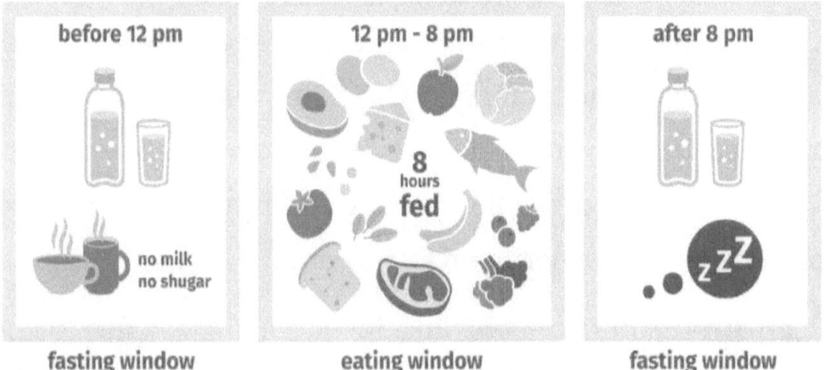

Intermittent fasting is just restricting your food to a certain period of time. There are several different types of IF to pick from. Choose the one that best matches your lifestyle, and then discuss it with the doctor.

1. Daily method. This is one of the most often used IF techniques. An 18/6 or 16/8 rule is often used in the daily method. This entails eating normal, nutritious things for six to eight hours each day and then fasting for the rest of 16 to 18 hours. This has been discovered as being the most long-term approach. To get started, experiment with different time options. A 12/12 diet involves eating for 12 hrs. and then fasting for twelve hours. When you're ready, you may go on to a more rigid timetable.

2. 5:2 method. This method entails eating regular, nutritious meals five days a week and restricting yourself to 500 to 600 calories two days a week. It's unclear if eating all of your calories in 1 sitting or spreading them out over the day is better, so do what suits you.

3. Alternate day method. You may eat regularly every other day if you select this technique. On fasting days, you'll consume just 25 percent of your daily calorie requirements. For instance, if you normally consume 1,800 calories per day, you will consume just 450 calories on fasting days.

4. 24-hour method. Fasting for a complete 24hrs before eating again is required for this strategy. Fasting from breakfast to the next breakfast or lunch to the next lunch is commonly done once or twice a week by those who utilize this strategy. If you utilize this strategy, proceed with care. It may cause extreme irritation, exhaustion, and headaches, and this way may or may not be beneficial for you.

2.4 Scientific Evidence about IF

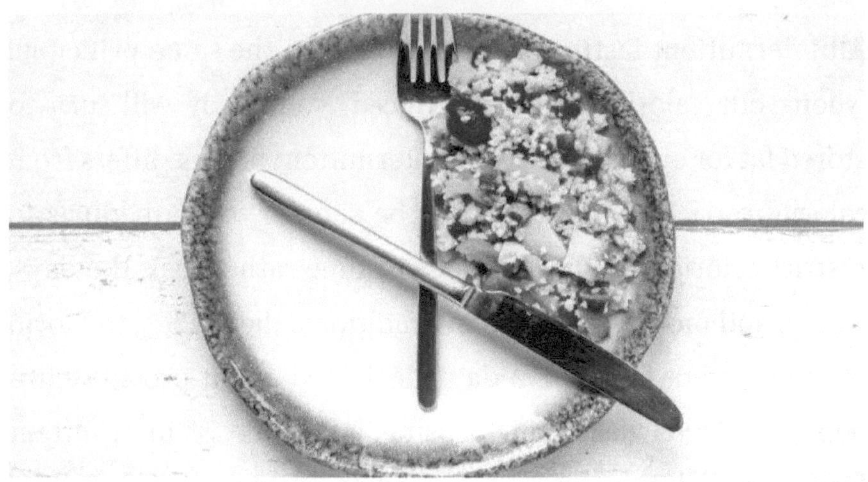

According to senior researcher Satchin Panda, although there is substantial scientific evidence for IF's advantages, it is neither a quick nor a definite remedy. A professor of circadian biology, Panda, at Salk Institute for Biological Studies in California, has dedicated his career to researching the human body's complicated biochemical processes. Intermittent fasting seems to boost human health in a number of ways, including weight loss, according to his study in mice and humans. Let's get one thing straight before you go into the science: Intermittent fasting may be done in a variety of ways. If you search it, you'll discover a slew of alternatives, each with its own set of supporters. The 5:2 diet entails eating extremely few calories (about 500-600) on 2 days of the week, then eating normally for five days. Alternate-day fasting is another option, which involves eating one day normally and then eating nothing or perhaps 500 calories the following.

All intermittent fasting strategies work on the same principle: when your calorie intake is reduced, your body will turn to stored fat for energy. However, intermittent fasting differs from calorie restriction in that it may be simpler for individuals to restrict calories for short periods of time rather than the days, weeks, and months required by traditional diets. Plus, the form of intermittent fasting Panda investigated might provide extra benefits. Panda has been focusing on a kind of intermittent fasting called time-restricted feeding. A person eats all of the calories for the day during an 8-to-12-hour span in this way. Let's pretend you start the day with a coffee cup at 7 a.m. and end it with popcorn & a drink at 11 p.m. You may change to eating breakfast at 8 a.m., including coffee, and completing your supper by 6 p.m. if you practice time-restricted eating. You'll be eating all of your meals inside a 10-hour timeframe, and you'll be skipping desserts, nighttime snacks, and alcohol calories. But it isn't the end of the narrative. Time-restricted eating appears to be beneficial to the body in more ways than just calorie reduction. Panda and colleagues' mouse research from 2012 was the first to propose this. They provided the same meal to two genetically identical pairs of mice, a lab-mice variant of the usual American diet, which is heavy in fat and simple sugar but low in protein.

While both of the groups were given an identical quantity of food, 1 group had access to it for 24 hours while the other only had access for 8 hours. Mice are nocturnal creatures that sleep during the daytime and feed at night. When one group of mice was given access to food 24 hours a day, they started consuming part of it while the day when they should have been sleeping. The mice that could feed at any time exhibited evidence of insulin resistance & liver damage after 18 weeks. These circumstances did not exist in the mice that ate within an 8-hour interval. They also weighed 28% less than mice that had access to food 24 hours a day, despite the fact that both the groups of mice consumed the same amount of calories each day. Panda says, "It was sort of earth-shattering." Until then, he and other academics believed that weight gain was governed by the overall quantity of calories consumed instead of when they were consumed. The experiment was repeated with three more groups of mice, and the findings were the same. The results were consistent across various kinds of food and feeding periods of up to 15 hours, albeit the shorter the window, the less weight the mice acquired. When time-restricted mice were given free rein for 2 days a week, or as Panda refers to as "taking the weekend off," they acquired less weight than mice that were permitted to eat 24 hours a day.

Panda's team next tried in another way: they swapped mice which had gained weight due to unlimited feeding for time-restricted eating. Despite ingesting the same number of calories, those mice dropped weight and kept it off for the duration of the research, which was 12 weeks. They also lowered insulin resistance, that is known to be connected to fat, but experts are still baffled by the relationship. Of course, the body of a human is more intricate than a mouse's, but these trials were the first hint of how crucial timing might be when it refers to how your bodies utilize food, according to Panda. Most of the human body's activities have been linked to circadian rhythms in recent years, according to experts. Most of you are aware that obtaining sunshine first thing in the morning is good for your mood and sleep, and being exposed to light after 9 p.m. through your mobile phones or computers may disturb your night's sleep. "Similarly, the correct food at the very right time may nourish you, whereas the wrong food at the wrong moment might be junk food," Panda explains. It is stored as fat instead of being utilized as fuel, which makes sense when you consider the foundations of human metabolism. Time-restricted eating allows your body to burn fat for longer periods of time. Your bodies utilize carbs for energy when you eat, and if you don't use them immediately away, they are stored as glycogen in the liver or turned into fat. Your bodies operate on glucose from carbs you've just eaten for some hours after you've done eating for a day before dipping into stored glycogen, or carbohydrates, in the liver. Your body's glycogen stores continue for many hours until running out about eight hrs. After you stop eating, at which point your bodies start to draw into their fat reserves. You spend more time in this fat-burning stage of your metabolism when you decrease your eating window & increase your fasting window. However, as soon as you consume food again, even if it's only a cup of coffee with a little sugar and milk, you revert to the opposite mode, burning carbs and storing glycogen & fat. So, if you complete your evening snack at 10 p.m., your body will run out of glycogen & begin burning fat at 6 a.m. If you modify your breakfast time from 6 a.m. to 9 a.m., you've given the body three more hours to burn fat for fuel.

Panda tested his time-restricted feeding trials on people and discovered that they were as promising. In 2015, he & his colleagues attempted to put a small sample of individuals on a 16-week time-restricted eating schedule. Surprisingly, the researchers provided these folks with no nutrition recommendations or instructions. Instead, the participants were instructed to eat just within a 10- to 12-hour timeframe. They snapped photographs of their meal and sent them to the researchers while they ate. The patients lost a little amount of weight, an average of slightly over 8 pounds apiece — after 16 weeks. According to Panda, they reported better sleep, greater energy in the mornings, and less hunger at night, indicating that time-restricted eating "really has a systemic influence all throughout the body." While the sample size was much too small to draw clear results, the researchers were encouraged that the modest intervention seemed to be straightforward for patients to execute and maintain. Time-restricted eating has been demonstrated to reduce the risk of diabetes. Panda and his colleagues discovered that after one week of restricting their meals to a nine-hour window, 15 men at risk for type-2 diabetes had a smaller jump in blood glucose following a test meal, indicating greater insulin sensitivity. It may also aid in the reduction of cholesterol. Panda and colleagues time-restricted the eating of 19 participants, the majority of whom were taking medication to decrease cholesterol, blood pressure, or diabetes. They reduced their overall cholesterol by roughly 11% on average after twelve weeks of eating within a 10-hour time frame. Panda then checked in a year later and discovered that around 34% of the individuals were still eating willingly in an 8 to 11-hour time frame. "It was great that they were able to self-sustain for such a long time," Panda adds. This is excellent news since,, according to some estimates, 13 to 12 percent of dieters gain back more bodyweight than they lost.

Time-restricted eating provides a number of benefits over other methods of weight loss: It's simple and straightforward. Diets are generally the luxury of those who can afford them since many individuals don't have time or means to count their calories, plan their meals, purchase particular foods, and monitor their calories. Anyone who can measure time & limit eating & drinking to specified intervals may practice time-restricted eating.

2.5 Intermittent Fasting Over other Diets

While most conventional diets include rules for what meals to eat and what foods to eliminate, one of the most tempting aspects of the Intermittent Fasting eating plan is that there are no foods that are forbidden. You may normally eat anything you want during the feasting period. Caloric restriction (& the advantages that come with it) may be achieved without having to give up meals you like.

There are many diets available, many of which claim to help people lose weight and stay healthy. Finding one that works might be difficult as a result. The IF diet is a trendy diet that has lately gained popularity. Most the traditional diets will include recommendations for which items to consume and which to avoid. The varieties of food that may be eaten on an IF diet is not limited. This is 1 of the reasons why some individuals find it more enticing. Let's see how intermittent fasting stacks up against some of the most popular diets.

Calories:

Many diets require people to monitor calories or at least think about how many calories they are consuming. It is feasible to consume the necessary quantity of calories on a time-restricted intermittent fasting regimen within the time limit that a person is permitted to eat. A person on a time-restricted IF diet will typically have a 6-8-hour window to eat. A regimen of alternate-day fasting indicates that a person would not eat at all on some days. This indicates that the calorie intake will fall short of the USDA's guidelines. Alternate-day fasting, on the other hand, is a superior strategy to reach weekly calorie objectives for persons who eat too many calories.

Variety:

One of the most appealing aspects of an IF diet is that it allows a person to eat anything they want. Intermittent fasting regimens do not contain suggested food categories, and participants are free to eat anything they choose. This differs from typical diets, which tend to limit some items while encouraging people to eat more of others. While this may be appealing to some, there is a disadvantage. There are usually no healthy food instructions included with an IF diet. This suggests that those who often consume processed meals are more inclined to do so in the future. A person who proceeds to eat a bad diet while sometimes fasting may not get the same health and weight-loss advantages as those who eat a healthy diet while fasting.

Convenience:

When it refers to dieting, the most common reason individuals fail is due to the diets they follow are just not suitable for their lifestyle. With IF, a person may still consume the things they want; the only restriction is the day or time they eat. For the most part, this makes the diet simple to follow. Other diets may include meal planning and grocery lists to find things easier to stick to. This might be a very smart approach to leading a healthy lifestyle for individuals who can regulate the quantity of food they consume. Overall, the fasting diets have shown potential, particularly for people who have difficulty sticking to a rigorous diet. It is crucial to remember, however, that fasting just for particular periods of time while continuing to make bad eating choices does not equate to a healthy lifestyle.

2.6 Combining IF with other Diets

Intermittent fasting is the practice of eating less often and reducing your eating window rather than a diet. You may combine intermittent fasting with whatever diet you desire, but you must avoid obsolete diets like low-fat or low-calorie diets and instead concentrate on consuming healthful foods and minimizing carbohydrates for the best results.

1. Keto Diet and Intermittent Fasting:

The keto diet (ketogenic) was created about a century ago to treat epilepsy in youngsters, and it has since acquired popularity owing to its effectiveness in weight reduction. The goal of this diet is to enter a state of ketosis. Ketosis occurs when your body switches from glycogen to ketone bodies as its principal source of energy. When you stop eating carbs, whether on a ketogenic diet or during a protracted fast, your metabolism changes. The ketogenic diet, according to a study, may offer a slew of health advantages.

- Type 2 diabetes, Obesity, and HDL cholesterol levels are some of the cardiovascular risk factors that may be improved. Although additional randomized controlled clinical trials are needed to offer precise recommendations, the ketogenic diet does have the potential to help treat several forms of cancer.

- When compared to high-carbohydrate diets, a low-carb diet improves glycemic control in people with type 2 diabetes.

- Diets with a low glycemic index, such as keto, are effective in treating epilepsy in patients of almost all ages.

- The advantages of the keto diet on polycystic ovarian syndrome have only been studied in a pilot study. Therefore additional research is needed. Low-carb diets, on the other hand, might be a potential therapy option for this ailment.

Combining the two:

Starting with a low-carb diet and adding IF protocols to your eating after a few weeks when the body is adapted to utilizing ketone bodies as its major source of energy is typical advice when combining Intermittent Fasting with the keto diet. Narrowing your eating windows & extending your fast times should be simpler when you're already in ketosis, according to IF plus keto experts. Mixing the two diets helps you lose weight because you are consuming fewer calories. You now not only eliminate an entire macro from your diet (because of keto), but you also miss dinners or breakfasts, depending on your IF program. Despite the fact that proponents of the ketogenic diet claim that this is not a calorie-counting diet, lowering your calorie intake aids weight reduction.

People Not Eligible for this Combination:

The primary disadvantage of combining IF with the ketogenic diet is how restricted it is. You constantly get advice that your diet must be sustainable when you speak about healthy weight reduction that you can maintain for the rest of your life. Rather than a short-term crash diet, you should make a long-term shift in your eating habits.

The keto diet has been more popular among individuals with type 2 diabetes or pre-diabetes since it has been shown to enhance glycemic control & even reduce medication use. Intermittent fasting, on the other hand, may increase the risk of hypoglycemia in people with type two diabetes. People who aren't a good match for intermittent fasting or keto diet should avoid combining the two. Intermittent fasting should not be attempted by anyone who has had or is currently experiencing eating disorders. Intermittent fasting is not recommended for pregnant or lactating women. Before starting intermittent fasting or keto diet programs, those with renal disease or any other health issues should see their doctors.

2. Intermittent Fasting and Mediterranean Diet:

The Mediterranean diet is mostly comprised of whole foods. It emphasizes the importance of fiber, plant foods, antioxidants, & healthy fats in one's diet. This is the usual Mediterranean diet (e.g., Greece, Spain, and Italy), and it is comparable to other diets that are plant-based such as pescatarian and flexitarian diets. The following foods should be included in your Mediterranean diet:

- Fruits of all kinds (frozen, fresh, dried)

- All of the veggies (fresh, dried, frozen, canned)

- Grain (whole), brown rice, bread, pasta, cereals, oats)

- Legume (beans, lentils, peas, chickpeas, soy)

- Seeds & nuts

- Spices & herbs

- As the main cooking oil, use olive oil (other examples of good vegetable oils are sesame, canola, walnut, and avocado oil)

- Seafood and fish (at least 2 times a week; fatty fish such as mackerel, salmon, and sardines are recommended)

- Eggs and poultry (small portions sometimes weekly, and white poultry meat is recommended)

- Dairy products with low fat (small portions sometimes a week)

- Meat that is low in fat (limited to some times per month)

Long-term adherence to a Mediterranean diet seems to be linked to the following health advantages:

- Type 2 diabetes risk is reduced.

- Metabolic syndrome risk is reduced.

- Metabolism-related diseases are less likely to occur.

- Depression, dementia, cognitive decline, and other mental diseases are all at a lower risk.

- Cholesterol balance

- Balance of blood pressure

- Cancer risk is reduced.

- Heart disease risk is reduced.

- BMI is lower.

- Getting to a healthy weight

- The body's Oxidative stress is reduced.

- Combining the two:

- You may profit from both a Mediterranean diet & an IF diet plan if you mix the two! The following is an example of a mixed eating plan:

- Following the Mediterranean diet by eating foods, snacks, meals, and drinks.

- Creating a "time-restricted eating" plan that fits your lifestyle

A time-restricted daily eating window of 8-12 hours seems to be a key component of this diet, according to evidence. With this in mind, combining the Mediterranean diet with 12 -16 hours of IF may be a healthy and sustainable diet choice with several health advantages. Other diets that may be used in conjunction with Intermittent Fasting include:

The Atkins diet, as the low-carb diet, when it comes to IF, is often suggested. They'll help you lose weight in a significant and long-term way if you combine them. A low-carb diet is a terrific strategy to reduce weight and has no health risks. And if you believe cutting carbohydrates is simpler than limiting the number of meals you eat, that's a great option for intermittent fasting. However, if you like a drink, chocolates with your coffee, bread, pizza, spaghetti, and other carb-heavy foods, intermittent fasting may be a better option. You may mix the two for maximum weight reduction or just lower carb consumption over time with IF. When you follow a fasting or low-carb diet, you'll notice certain cravings (sugar, carbohydrates), and your hunger will decrease.

Paleo, like a low-carb diet, maybe a perfect supplement to intermittent fasting, and it offers some of the same advantages as IF, such as lower insulin resistance, blood pressure, and triglycerides. Intermittent fasting is enhanced by a low-carb diet supplemented with healthful items. It will assist you in losing weight and improving your overall health. Paleo will limit your food options, but it should be simpler to stick to than Keto or even Atkins diet. It is still a certain technique to reduce weight, break your sugar addiction, and so on. It all relies on your own preferences and what you're willing to give up in order to better your health. Implementing a mild version of the Paleo diet, allowing for a few beers on weekends and the odd pizza with friends while intermittent fasting, might be a terrific approach to losing weight and forming healthy habits over time without going all in.

The Carnivore Diet is an absolute no-carb diet, so it fits nicely in with fasting. However, this is such a specialized, restricted diet, and the research on the effect of this sort of diet is so limited that you must only undertake it if you have all of the facts. That isn't a magic cure-all diet. Yes, you'll be eliminating all carbohydrates, which may assist with a variety of ailments, but you'll also be consuming a very restricted diet. Although it has been claimed that animal-sourced food contains the majority of nutrients, no significant research has been undertaken to prove that it is a safer diet to follow. The carnivore diet isn't so much about losing weight as it is about improving or curing specific illnesses. It should also be looked at and explored in light. Fasting has a broad list of advantages, and some of the side effects of turning carnivorous (sugar addiction, health problems) may be alleviated by simple intermittent fasting (IF) or even longer fasts.

2.7 Benefits for Women over 50

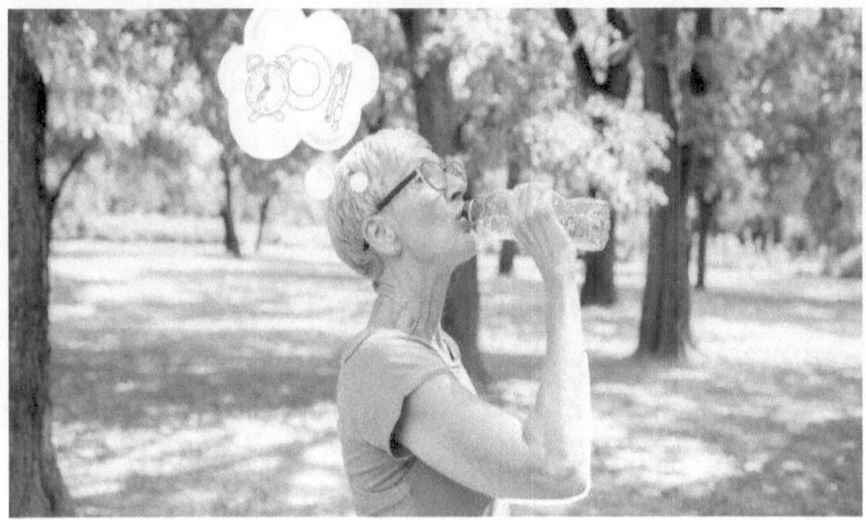

Weight reduction is a well-known IF advantage. When you consume all of the calories in a short period of time, you eat less overall. There will be less weight gain if you consume less. In addition to weight reduction, intermittent fasting also has the following benefits:

- Encourages ketosis (ketosis helps you with hunger management & mental acuity)

- It has been shown that it improves cardiovascular risk indicators.

- Could aid in the reversal of type 2 diabetes

- Aids in the enhancement of your circadian rhythm, or 24-hour wake-sleep cycle.

- Aids in the activation of autophagy, a cellular longevity function.

Both pre-menopausal & post-menopausal women have benefited from intermittent fasting. In one research, 75 obese men & women over the age of 50 were given alternate-day fasting (ADF). Participants ate five hundred calories on fasting days & as much as they wanted on non-fasting days for a period of 12 weeks. On average, everyone benefitted, regardless of menopausal status or sex. Fat mass, insulin resistance, fasting insulin, and blood pressure were all reduced in all groups. Interestingly, postmenopausal women had lower LDL cholesterol (a risk factor for heart disease) than premenopausal women. Another study looked at a sort of fasting known as time-restricted feeding (TRF). TRF entails eating all of the daily calories in a short period of time. Obese women in the research ate for 8 weeks within a 4-6 hour eating window. This is halfway between 16/8 & OMAD (1 (one) meal a day) for those acquainted with IF procedures. The findings were comparable to those of the earlier research. Pre-menopausal and post-menopausal women both dropped weight and improved their metabolic health. These are desired advantages for women beyond the age of 50. Post-menopausal women are more likely to gain weight, develop cardiovascular disease, and have problems controlling their blood sugar levels due to estrogen deficiency. Intermittent fasting diets aren't all created with weight reduction in mind.

Detoxification, blood sugar stabilization, blood pressure control, hormone regulation, and decreased inflammation are some of the additional health advantages of intermittent fasting. One of the main reasons for women over 50 to pursue intermittent fasting is to get greater energy. Many women report a small weight increase and worse sleep quality as they approach menopause. Both of these things might make you sleepy and sluggish. However, you may retrain your body to feel better by modifying when & what you consume. Other IF advantages for women over 50 include:

Anti-Aging:

As you become older, wrinkles occur, unexpected aches and pains arise, and you go through the emotional shifts that come with growing older. Intermittent fasting provides a number of anti-aging advantages. Every year, women spend hundreds of dollars on lotions & potions to turn the clock back. Intermittent fasting may provide the same results at no cost. Women's bodies naturally limit the production of HgH (Human Growth Hormone), sometimes known as the "fountain of youth," as they become older. This "fountain of youth" may be triggered by intermittent fasting.

Relieve joint discomfort:

According to a 2016 research published in the Journal of Mid-Life Health, fasting helps decrease joint discomfort, which prevents some women from getting the activity they need to sustain their long-term weight reduction outcomes.

It alleviates anxiety and despair:

In addition, many women over 50 suffer from anxiety and/or depression and are often administered drugs that cause weight gain as a side effect. The same research found that when women in their forties and fifties fast on a regular basis, their anxiety and sadness levels drop. IF is the ideal lifestyle for women over 50, & it may provide the groundwork for a long, healthy, and happy life. If you're worried about menopause, you can be interested to discover that IF can get you through it.

Metabolic Health:

Menopause strikes some women in their fifties. Menopause affects a woman's body in a number of ways, including a reduction in muscle mass, metabolism, and hormonal changes. For women over 50, intermittent fasting may help lower belly fat, blood pressure, and cholesterol levels while also boosting insulin sensitivity. Fasting may also aid in the regulation and tracking of the metabolism as you become older.

Energy levels have been improved.

When you aren't continually digesting meals throughout the day, you have more energy to do other things. After transitioning to intermittent fasting, many women over 50 years of age report having consistent energy levels throughout the day. The ability to no longer feel peaks & troughs in energy levels may be a liberating feeling.

Insulin resistance is reduced.

Intermittent fasting has indeed been demonstrated to enhance insulin sensitivity and regulate blood sugar levels. When women eat in this manner, they have been able to reverse type 2 diabetes. Insulin resistance is widespread in men and women over the age of 50, but it doesn't have to really be an inevitable part of the aging process.

Musculoskeletal health has improved.

Arthritis, Osteoporosis, and lower back discomfort are all examples of this. Fasting has been found to increase thyroid hormone output. This may help avoid bone fractures by promoting bone health.

IF has also been shown to have the following advantages:

- Memory enhancement

- Tissue well-being

- Physical abilities

- Improves Heart health.

2.8 Potential Risks & People not Eligible

Most women seem to be safe when using modified variants of intermittent fasting. On the other hand, a series of research have shown that fasting days might cause hunger, mood changes, loss of focus, decreased energy, headaches, and foul breath. Women's menstrual cycles have also been reported to have ceased while on an intermittent fasting diet, according to some reports on the internet. Before attempting intermittent fasting, ask your doctor if you have a medical issue.

- Women who have a past of eating problems should seek medical advice immediately.

- Have diabetes or encounter low levels of blood sugar on a frequent basis.

- Are underweight, malnourished, or deficient in nutrients.

- Expecting a child, nursing, or trying to conceive

- Ever had reproductive issues or a past of amenorrhea (missed periods).

- Finally, intermittent fasting seems to have a favorable safety profile. However, if you have any issues, such as a lack of your menstrual period, you should stop immediately.

University of Illinois researchers found, "Intermittent fasting is typically safe and does not cause a decline in energy level changes or enhanced disordered eating habits." However, they cautioned that this dietary regimen is not suitable for all women over the age of 50. Those with a past of unhealthy eating, a BMI of less than 18.5, or those that need to take medicine with meals at regular intervals should avoid it. People with specific medical issues, according to some specialists, may not be good candidates. Women suffering from Crohn's disease, for example, may benefit from a modified diet. Those with diabetes usually are advised to avoid it, particularly if their blood sugar levels aren't adequately managed. Fasting on a regular basis isn't for everyone. Always check with your physician before starting a brand new diet, even if it has been demonstrated to be helpful. The following mentioned groups of persons should be avoided in general IF:

- Children under eighteen years of age

- People who have had an eating issue in the past

- Women who are pregnant or nursing

Chapter 3: Journey of Intermittent Fasting – The Best Way to do it

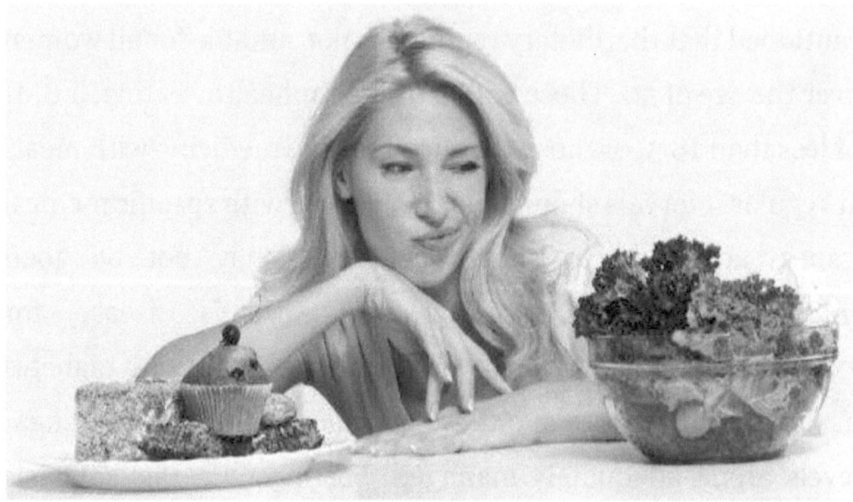

Some individuals may leap directly into intermittent fasting by flipping a switch, while others must gradually change their eating habits. You're in a world that's been overfed. It may take some time to adjust to eating less since it is ingrained in our psychology to have a large breakfast and nibble throughout the day. Perhaps you'll begin intermittent fasting on Mondays, Wednesdays, and Fridays or simply on weekends. Whatever method works best for you to begin.

3.1 Step by Step Process

For starters, Greaves, an expert, says IF isn't for women who don't get enough sleep, don't eat enough or regularly, have irregular or nonexistent periods, have thyroid difficulties, have a history of present or former disordered eating, are below a lot of stress, or have blood sugar problems. Start slowly if your doctor or nutritionist has given you permission. "Some studies have indicated that fasting for 12 - 14 hours overnight just may result in metabolic improvements," Greaves notes. "It's essential to realize that you don't have to keep fast for 16 /18 hours to get the benefits." She advocates beginning with the time-restricted strategy rather than the 5:2 method, which limits calories two days a week while encouraging patients to gorge on the other days.

To begin, determine how many hours it takes you to go from the time you finish eating at night to the time you begin eating the following day. To begin, broaden your fast by 1 hour, then two hours, and so on. There are no calorie limitations with time-restricted IF. It is suggested to eat three balanced meals a day, spread equally during the eating window, with protein, high-fiber carbs, and healthy fats. Those who've never been huge breakfast eaters might find it simple to wait until 10 or 11 a.m. to eat, while others wake up ravenous. An essential thing is to pay attention to the body and eat when hungry. Intermittent fasting may be challenging for women who exercise often. It will be difficult to fast if it is that phase of the month & you are hungry.Can coffee help you break your fast? Yes, technically, if there's something in it. There are no calories in black coffee. But think about your objectives: are you trying to lose weight? If that's the case, keep in mind that IF doesn't cause any more loss of weight than a calorie deficit, so a little creamer in your coffee is probably safe. Are you doing this to keep your blood sugar in check? If that's the case, then a caramel latte isn't the ideal way to begin the day. The overall procedure would be as follows:

Step 1: Cut the Breakfast Out

Breakfast is an essential meal of the day. The simplest and most effective approach to begin IF is to eliminate breakfast from your daily routine. In the morning, your body does its own miracle. It is only interrupted by food. In the morning, cortisol hormones & adrenals rise to help you get up, become aware, and produce energy.

Step 2: Determine When the Ideal Time to Exercise Is

Many people believe they can't exercise while fasting, although the contrary is true. The finest time for strong exercise is in the morning! You're young and healthy, with hormonal balance on your side. Afternoon and evening exercises aren't always as successful as they may be; you're exhausted from the day, preoccupied with whatever new pressures have thrown at you at work, and resisting the impulse to kick off your shoes and relax.

Step 3: Unwind. Your (unsweetened) coffee is still safe to drink!

Yes! Fortunately for coffee enthusiasts worldwide, your beloved morning ritual does neither raise blood sugar nor cause a fast to be broken. If you can't stand the thought of drinking black coffee, add some creamer... However, not too much! Remember that your body must burn the fat in creamer just before it can return to burning the stored fat. What about coffee consumers who require a sweetener to conceal bitterness? All-natural sweeteners, such as honey, cane sugar, and agave nectar, should be avoided, according to Zane, an expert on intermittent fasting. Although they are "natural" carbohydrates, they spike blood sugar & insulin levels almost instantly. As a result, your body will no longer be in a fasting state. Stick to a modest dash of Stevia in your coffee if you want a bit of sweetness. The majority of artificial sugars are harmful because they trigger cravings and deceive the digestive system into anticipating sugar that will never arrive. This messes with the fat-burning mechanism that fasting is supposed to help with. In the end, the issue of coffee comes down to your objectives. If you're trying to lose fifty pounds, putting cream on your daily coffee may stymie your efforts. A sugary cup of coffee, on the other hand, is much superior to a piece of cheesecake! It's all about striking the right balance.

Step 4: This Is Also For Diabetics!

Zane (an expert on IF) deals with diabetic customers on a daily basis who feel intermittent fasting is too dangerous. "I don't know of a better method to regulate diabetes or cure those symptoms than figuring out a way to introduce fasting," he says. Type two diabetes is a blood sugar imbalance illness, and IF is a powerful tool for lowering and balancing blood sugar levels via healthier eating habits. Fasting is the most effective tool for improving glycemic control. Diabetics can be able to utilize fasting to remove their need for medication and lessen the consequences of diabetes if they follow a deliberate, doctor-guided approach.

Step 5: Plan Your Lunch and Dinner around Your Fasting Routines

You've had your share of information and are ready to enter into the lovely world of IF. So, when are you allowed to eat? "The easiest approach...is to forgo breakfast and have coffee or tea instead," Zane explains. "Eat a low-carb lunch & supper if you want to lose weight." After the fasting window expires, you eat your 1st meal of the day, which means you consume all of your meals inside a six to eight-hour window. "It's a give-and-take situation." Make sure it fits into your schedule. If it's six hours, that's fantastic. "Don't beat yourself up if it must be 9 one day," Zane adds.

The beauty of IF is that there is no wrong or right way to do it. It's one tool you can use to enhance your health in whichever manner works best for you. Here's what you can do for a good intermittent fasting schedule:

- After supper, you should stop eating (8:00 PM)

- Fast till midday, skipping breakfast and enjoying a cup of black coffee or tea.

- A low-carb meal can help you break your fast.

- If you must have a snack, keep it light.

- Enjoy a hearty supper before resuming your fast.

- Once you've become used to the pattern of intermittent fasting, try extending your fast till one, two, or three a.m. instead.

Step 6: Get Involved With the Dinnertime Community

There's a reason why most individuals choose to forego breakfast over supper. Your evening meals are social and interpersonal in nature. That's how it's been for millennia! You use supper to unwind from the day, reconcile with family, and commemorate the passing of another day. You don't have to miss out on such a rewarding experience. Instead, use the time to develop mindfulness while eating. You'll enjoy every piece of your dinner much more than if you'd been nibbling all day. Fasting is most effective when you retain supper as your primary meal relationship, as Zane observes with his clients.

Step 7: Consume for a Reason

When it comes to intermittent fasting, you need to figure out when to open your mouth. But what should you consume

after you've opened your mouth? There is no one-size-fits-all solution; it all relies on your objectives.

- If you're trying to Lose Weight.

If you're trying to lose pounds, it is suggested to decrease your carbohydrate and sugar intake. Make it as simple as possible by arranging the meal you'll eat to break the fast each day. Preparing a filling, low-carb lunch can help you avoid making rash judgments. Dinner should consist of a lean protein & a vegetable, although a healthy carbohydrate or fat is OK. Remember: You're rewarding yourself with healthful, enjoyable meals, not punishing yourself!

- If losing weight isn't your primary goal.

Focus on consuming actual things if you're fasting for health and longevity's sake. It would not be food now if it wasn't food 100 years ago! To escape the unseen trap of added sugars, avoid packaged, processed foods and read labels. It's important to find a good combination of healthy fats, proteins and fruits and vegetables. You'll immediately restrict your consumption of those sneaky carbs if you eat these actual meals.

Step 8: One day a week, try a 24-hour fast.

Don't get too worked up over the 24-hr fast. Once you've become used to intermittent fasting, switching to a 24-hour fast once a week isn't such a huge deal. After supper is the best time to begin a 24-hour fast. Instead of ending your fast at 1:00 p.m.

with lunch, wait a few hours and break it with supper and celebration. Fasting 1 day a week, the first meal following a 24-hr fast, is really gratifying. It's unlike anything else. Not to consider the fat-burning and metabolic advantages of a 24-hour body reset.

Step 9: Say No to a Cheat Day during Intermittent Fasting

For most individuals, a cheat day is equal to a binge day, except the consequences of the binge don't go away after 24 hours. To heal from the impacts of a cheat day, rein in your desires, restore your energy and attention, and come back on track, it might take 3 or 4 days. "Why throw it all over with a complete plate of pizza or a lot of pancakes if your aim is weight reduction and you're trying to go there effectively? During an IF cheat day, a spike of 1,500 caloric intake of junk food will send you in the reverse way of your objectives. An indulgence, on the other hand, is a different matter. A slice of pie or a few cookies every now and then may aid you in scratching an urge before it becomes a rash that causes you to get stranded.

3.2 Choosing Best Pattern to Assist your Purpose

Intermittent fasting may be done in a number of ways. Among the most famous are:

- the method of 16:8

- Eat Stop Eat

- the Warrior diet

- Fasting on alternating days (ADF)

- the 5:2 eating plan

All strategies may be helpful, but determining which one works best for you is a personal decision. Here's a rundown of the benefits and drawbacks of each strategy to help you decide which is best for you.

The method of 16/8:

One of the most popular fasting plans for weight reduction is the 16/8 IF strategy. Food & calorie-containing drinks are restricted to an 8-hr. window each day below the diet. It necessitates fasting for remaining of 16 hrs. of day. Whilst other diets might have severe regulations and restrictions, the 16/8 method is easy and its basis is on a TRF (time-restricted feeding) concept. You may eat calories on any 8-hour period. Some individuals refrain from eating late and follow a 9 a.m. to 5 p.m. schedule, whereas others skip breakfast & fast from 12 p.m. to 8 p.m. Limiting the amount of hours you may eat throughout the day will help you lose weight and lower your blood pressure. According to studies, time-restricted eating patterns, like the 16/8 method, may help people avoid hypertension and eat less, resulting in weight reduction. When combined with weight exercise, the 16/8 method was shown to efficiently decrease fat mass while retaining muscle mass in men in a 2016 research.

A more recent research found that the 16/8 method had no effect on muscle or strength gains in women who completed resistance training. While the 16/8 technique may easily be adopted into any routine, some individuals may find going 16 hrs. without eating challenging. Furthermore, eating too many junk food or snacks during the 8-hr. fasting window might negate the 16/8 intermittent fasting advantages. Consume a healthy diet rich in fruits, whole grains, vegetables, healthy fats, and protein to gain the maximum health advantages from this diet.

The 5:2 method:

The 5:2 method is a simple intermittent fasting strategy. You consume regularly for five days a week and don't count your calories. Then you restrict your calorie intake to one-quarter of the everyday requirements on other 2 days of week. For a person who eats 2k calories each day on a regular basis, this will entail restricting their calorie intake to 500 calories 2 days every week. The 5:2 diet is equally as beneficial as the daily calorie restriction for the reduction of weight and blood glucose management among people with type 2 diabetes, as per a 2018 study. Another research indicated that in people with type 2 diabetes, the 5:2 diet is equally as effective as daily restriction of calorie for weight reduction and blood glucose management. Another research found that this diet was equally as effective as constant calorie restriction for weight reduction and the avoidance of metabolic diseases including diabetes and heart disease. On full-calorie days, the 5:2 diet enables you to pick which days you want to fast, and that there are no limitations on when or what you eat.

It's important to note, though, that eating "normally" on full-calorie days doesn't mean you can eat everything you want. It's tough to restrict oneself to five hundred calories a day, even if it's just for days a week. Additionally, consuming too little calories might make you feel ill or faint. The 5:2 diet may be useful for some people, but it isn't for everyone. To find out whether this diet is right for you, go to your doctor.

Eat Stop Eat:

Brad Pilon, writer of "Eat Stop Eat," promoted an innovative intermittent fasting strategy known as "Eat Stop Eat." This approach of intermittent fasting comprises selecting on 1 or 2 non-consecutive days each week when you will fast for 24 hours. The remainder of the week is yours to eat whatever you like, but it's ideal to eat a healthy well-balanced diet & avoid overindulging. The notion that consuming fewer calories would result in weight reduction justifies a weekly 24-hour fast.

Fasting for straight 24 hours might cause a metabolic shift, leading your body to use fat as an energy source rather than glucose. However, fasting for 24 hrs. at a time requires a great deal of self-control and may lead to bingeing & overeating afterwards. It might also lead to a change in eating habits. More study is required to determine this diet's potential health benefits and weight reduction properties. Consult your doctor before beginning Eat Stop Eat to see whether it's a healthy weight-loss strategy for you.

Alternate-day fasting

A basic, easy-to-follow IF diet is alternate-day fasting. On this diet, you fast every alternate day but eat anything you like on the non-fasting days. Some forms of this diet use a "modified" fasting strategy that involves ingesting around 500 calories on fasting days. On the other hand, some variations totally exclude calories on the fasting days. People who fast on alternate days have been demonstrated to lose weight. Alternate-day fasting was shown to be as effective for weight reduction as calorie restriction in a randomised pilot study of obese persons. Another research found that people consumed 35 percent less calories & lost an almost of 3.5 kg (7.7 pounds) after switching between 36 hrs. and 12 hours of fasting of unrestricted eating for 4 weeks . Incorporating an exercise programme into your everyday routine will help you lose weight if you're serious about losing weight. Combining this fasting with endurance exercise, according to study, may result in weight reduction that is twice as effective as merely fasting.

Fasting for one whole day every second day might be difficult, particularly if you're new to it. It's easy to overindulge on non-fasting days. Start with a modified fasting schedule to ease into this method of fasting if you're new to intermittent fasting. Whether you start with a limited fasting plan or a complete fast, it's best to eat a well-balanced meal that includes high-protein foods and low-calorie veggies to keep you feeling full.

The Warrior diet

This Diet is a strategy inspired by old warriors' eating habits. The Warrior Diet, developed by Ori Hofmekler in 2001, is more intense than the 16:8 technique but less restricted than Eat Fast Eat method. It includes eating relatively little all through the day for 20 hrs. and then eating as much as you wanted during the 4-hr window at the night. During the 20-hr. fast, this diet advises dieters to eat tiny quantities of raw fruits, hard-boiled eggs,

dairy products, and vegetables, and also non-calorie drinks. After a 20-hr, fast, people may eat anything they like during a 4-hour window, however unprocessed, nutritional, and natural meals are recommended. While no studies on the Warrior Diet have been conducted, human studies have indicated that time-restricted food cycles may lead to weight reduction. There are no other recognised health advantages of time-restricted eating cycles. TRF cycles have been demonstrated to reduce diabetes, slow tumour growth, and lengthen longevity in mice. To fully appreciate the Warrior Diet's weight-loss advantages, further study is required.

Because the Warrior Diet restricts calorie consumption to just 4 hours each day, it may be difficult to keep to. Overeating at night time is a common occurrence. Eating problems have been related to the Warrior Diet. Whether you're up to the challenge, talk to your doctor to see if it's suitable for you.

3.3 The Right Mindset to Start

It appears to be common knowledge that everything boils down to discipline and adhering to the "no pain, no gain" philosophy. You forget that your bodies aren't machines when you think like this. Your bodies cease working correctly as a result of all the stress you put on yourself. The solution is the appropriate frame of mind! When it refers to reducing weight, stress is the greatest deterrent. According to studies, too much stress might prevent fat burning. This is mostly due to stress chemicals produced, such as cortisol, which inhibits fat metabolism. But you have the power to alter your mental state! You have the power to affect and change it - if you so want! Now is the time to change your thinking; it may take some time, but it is vitally important to remember these things:

1. Make an invitation to your body.

2. Don't try to oppose it.

3. Develop the ability to pay attention to your body's requirements. Patience is required.

4. Recognize and respect your limitations; don't push yourself too much if you don't feel like it.

Everything changes once you end up thinking of your body as an adversary! Many things get simpler right away when you work with them rather than against them. If you want to cultivate a good mindset, IF may assist you:

Intermittent fasting may aid in the development of a more cheerful attitude. Fasting on a regular basis enhances your connection with food (and also with yourself).

- You relearn how to attend to your own needs.

- You grow more conscious and autonomous by removing yourself from the steady stream of consumption.

- While fasting, you give the body the time & space it needs to recuperate and renew.

Weight loss doesn't really have to be a struggle. The secret to your success has the appropriate mentality and attitude. It takes time to change your thinking. If you find yourself reverting to old habits, don't become discouraged. Keep a good attitude and keep going - even if you're intermittent fasting! After some time, you'll notice that it happens less often. Every step you take gets you nearer to your objective.

3.4 S.M.A.R.T Way – Set Achievable Goals

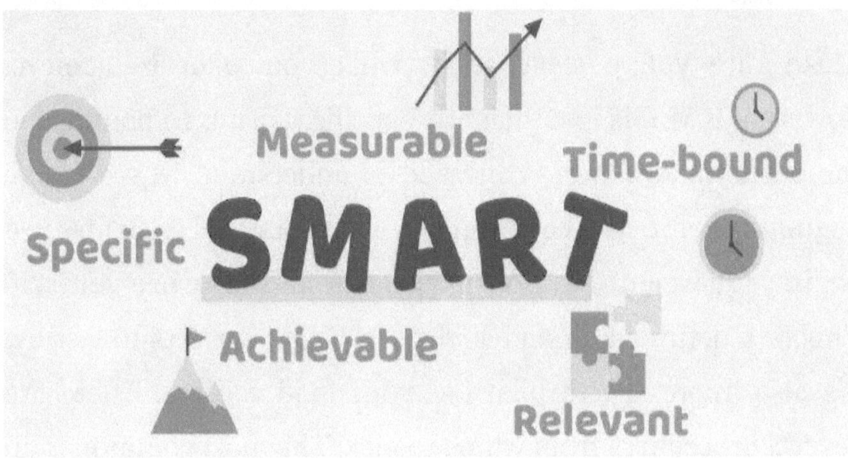

'It is believed that almost 44 million Americans strive to reduce weight each year, according to statistics polls. According to another research, 38 percent of Americans have attempted to lose more weight than three times. These results reveal a few things: weight loss is difficult, and many of you don't know how to accomplish it properly. S.M.A.R.T. (Specific Measurement and Reporting Techniques) is a framework for defining goals. It may be used in every aspect of your life, but it is extremely beneficial for weight reduction. When paired with intermittent fasting, this strategy may be incredibly practical and simple to follow. Setting these goals and pairing them with IF (meal timing) can get you nearer to your target weight quicker than you think. Furthermore, weight reduction outcomes acquired using this strategy are more certain to last than those obtained in a chaotic manner without any structure. Here's how to use the S.M.A.R.T. goal-setting system to help you lose weight.

Specific:

Make sure you're clear about what you want to achieve. Lowering B.M.I. is insufficiently specific. Losing 10 pounds, on the other hand, is not. You need to understand where you're beginning before you can establish what your goal is. Before you begin your weight-loss journey, weigh and measure yourself. Choose a definite aim and stick to it. When it refers to fasting, it's also important to plan out your food routine. There are several procedures from which to pick. The most common is an 8-hr eating window followed by a 16-hour fast.

Starting slowly and having a 14-hr eating window is a great choice also if this sounds too hard. Males are advised to use the 16:8 approach. However, ladies may safely use the 14:10 schedule.

Measurable:

You must be able to track your progress in order to attain your objective. This implies that if you don't have a device to track your steps, you shouldn't set a target of 10,000 steps. It may be difficult to keep track of health indicators on your own, so having a physician examine you is a good option. Find out how you're doing in terms of your health, and then work with your doctor to create clear, quantifiable objectives. Repeat the tests the next time you've got an appointment, and you'll be able to see how far you've progressed.

Remember to be precise. If you are going to be fasting, a medical evaluation is very important. Eating within certain time frames has health advantages that are difficult, if not impossible, to quantify with the naked eye. Before you begin, you may want to know what proportion of your body fat is visceral. Set a target to shed at least 1 percent of the dangerous fat that surrounds your organs, and be sure to check in with your doctor to see whether you've met it.

Attainable:

It is critical to ensure that a goal is attainable while establishing one. Of course, reducing 50 pounds with a one-meal-a-day fasting program sounds like a worthwhile objective, but think about whether you will be able to stick to the schedule for long enough. Unrealistic objectives might soon dissuade you from making any kind of strategy at all. Instead, start modest, and you'll be able to change your objective at any time. Start with 2 pounds if you need to shed 100 pounds. Alternatively, if you're not sure whether you should start, make a list of the benefits and drawbacks of intermittent fasting. Small objectives are both feasible and encouraging to achieve.

Relevant:

When deciding on a goal, consider if it is meaningful to your life. When you achieve your objective, what you do and how you do it will change. What personal significance does this aim have for you? The good news is that any weight-loss-related objectives are typically quite relevant to the individual who is attempting to attain them. Weight loss translates to improved self-esteem, health, more bonding time with your friends & family, and less frustration, among other benefits. After a setback, whatever significance you assign to your objective will aid you in getting back on track. If you don't know why you are losing weight or if you're content with your current weight, you're unlikely to achieve your weight reduction goals. Simply said, it has no bearing on you. Relevant goal-setting example: "I'll feel more energized after I start an IF program and drop 10 pounds. More clothing that fits me will be available to me. My health would improve, and I'll have more time to spend with my grandkids."

Time-bound:

Consider that if a goal doesn't have a deadline, it isn't a goal at all. You must be able to achieve your objective within a certain amount of time. It is advisable for a beginning 'goal setter' to establish short-term objectives. Set daily or weekly objectives for intermittent fasting & weight reduction, pay close attention to all of the previously mentioned information and make adjustments as needed. Like "Set an objective to lose 1 pound in 1 week (time-bound) while implementing a 16:8 IF routine" Knowing that you can achieve your objectives will make you feel better about yourself. It will assist you in developing new weight-loss strategies (relevant). To get the greatest outcomes, you will change your objectives on a weekly basis."

3.5 Monitoring Your Progress and Self-Motivation

Because IF has a unique method for tackling weight loss & energy generation, it may be tough to track your success if you're new to it. However, there are a few ways to detect when Intermittent Fasting begins to work & monitor your progress if you're new to it.

1. You Aren't Hungry

Intermittent fasting decreases hunger by boosting lipolysis, a fat-burning mechanism. (1) It aids in the fat-burning process by enabling the fat-storing hormone insulin to naturally drop during a fasting condition. This fat-burning mechanism supplies the body with a consistent energy supply, signaling to your body that it doesn't need to eat.

2. Body Fat Percentage Is Declining

Intermittent Fasting largely utilizes fat as fuel, according to a 2020 review of IF and weight reduction. Intermittent fasting is particularly unusual in that it has been shown to stimulate muscle-protecting hormones like growth hormones naturally. This combination promotes fat burning while preserving muscular mass.

3. Reduced Bloating and Improved Bowel Movements

Intermittent fasting has another effect that is frequently overlooked or overlooked: it stimulates the gut cleansing process known as the MMC (Migrating Motor Complex). It is only activated when you don't eat (called fasting), and it helps to flush away leftover food and germs that cause bloating. The MMC may be stimulated by adopting Intermittent Fasting.

4. Increased Energy Levels

Intermittent fasting induces cellular cleansing, known as autophagy, which is one of its most well-known benefits. This procedure eliminates faulty mitochondria & cells that are inefficient in generating energy. This cleansing process allows more high-performing cells & mitochondria to grow, resulting in more consistent energy levels. Not to add that increased fat metabolism (fat decomposition) offers a more dependable energy source than glucose.

5. Sugar Cravings are reduced

Sugar cravings are reduced as a result of the increased fat-burning processes associated with Intermittent Fasting. Sugar cravings are mostly physiological in nature. It's usually a symptom that you didn't consume enough fat/protein at your previous meal or that your body is dependent on sugar/glucose for energy. During the fasting phase, switching to fat as a fuel source may assist in significantly decreasing sugar cravings. The only exception is if you are opening your fast with a high-sugar/starch meal, which will swiftly derail your Intermittent Fasting outcomes.

Self-Motivation- Some useful tips:

Fasting has several advantages. However, just because you understand all of the advantages of a healthier life doesn't imply you will be able to remain motivated to follow it all of the time. The tactics listed below may help you become and remain motivated. You are not obligated to use just 1 of these motivating techniques. In fact, by using a mix of them, you'll have a better chance of succeeding. Find out which ones are best for you and put them into practice.

Look for a fasting accountability partner.

Enlisting a companion, or an accountability buddy, to help you in a journey of healthy lifestyle makeovers has been found to increase your chances of success. You'll lose more weight and stick to the diet for a long time than if you tried it on your own. The companion you choose doesn't necessarily have to be local in today's world of global connectivity. Perhaps a Facebook buddy from across the nation wishes to join in this new lifestyle, or you'd like to join an internet forum or group.

Watch videos or read articles/blogs.

To become or remain inspired, all you have to do is watch or read anything that inspires you. Reading a blog or many articles on someone else's great body and lifestyle transformations, or seeing a video clip about somebody's successful body & lifestyle transformations, maybe highly motivating and help you feel up to the challenge of adhering to your new healthy lifestyle.

Make a short-term objective with a monetary incentive.

Choose a target which you can measure & achieve in a reasonable length of time, and once you've accomplished it, treat yourself to something that isn't linked to junk food, like a massage or new training gear. Though food is your ultimate reward, you will continuously feel as if you are starving yourself when you aren't consuming certain items. Instead, select a prize that is significant to you but does not need you to sabotage your success.

Recognize when a carrot is required and when a stick is required.

Rewarding yourself might not be quite as effective at keeping you motivated as "punishing" yourself for not achieving a goal. Eating correctly, fasting, exercising properly, and so on are not penalties when it comes to living a healthy lifestyle. You may have already spent years believing that they are, & you need to entirely change your mind.

Be truthful to yourself.

Shut your eyes and envision what your life would be like in the future, 3, 6 or 12 months or more, if you stopped today. Make sure you're being completely honest with yourself. Create questions and situations based on how you felt & looked before you started your healthy living journey, as well as the positive improvements you've seen thus far. This motivating technique pushes you to reflect on your life before resolving to become healthy, as well as how much terrible you will feel if you stay down that unhealthy road. That future may be a frightening place, but the wonderful thing about it is that it hasn't yet been chosen.

Visualize yourself in a healthy state in the future.

If you stick to your present healthy lifestyle makeover, you may utilize visualization to visualize and imagine what a healthy future would look like. With visualization, you reproduce all of the visuals, sensations, and even noises of a certain event, but you only allow for a good conclusion, excluding any negative sentiments or ideas that may otherwise prevent you from succeeding.

Concentrate on the good sensations.

Self-assured, balanced, energized, and alive. Have any of these pleasant sensations come to you when you first began fasting? If you're seeking inspiration, go back to when you first started your health journey and recall how fantastic you felt about this new lifestyle. Maybe just after successfully finishing a fast or refusing dessert, or after getting a remark on your gorgeous complexion, or after waking up for the 1st time in years feeling completely rested. Knowing that you had finished a day-long fast made you feel fantastic.

Make a list of the good things that have happened to you.

You might not be able to notice the progress you've already made since you're in the middle of things. If that's the case, instead of focusing on the progress you haven't achieved, take stock of the good improvements you've seen while committing to a fasting approach (yet). Take note of how much more comfortable your clothing fit. Consider how well you've been sleeping recently.

Self-compassion is important.

You won't always feel inspired, and you won't always have as productive a day or 1 week as you'd want. Negative self-talk and beating yourself up because you didn't reach your own standards won't benefit you in the long term. When you're going through a tough period, the greatest thing you may do is be kind to yourself.

Make it a habit to motivate oneself.

Motivation is more likely a habit, and as with all habits, it must be practiced in order to become second nature. And put it into practice on a routine basis. Set aside 15 - 20 minutes each day to reflect on your objectives, progress, where you are now, & where you want to go. Find relevant positive affirmations and say them to yourself – in your head, in the vehicle, or in front of the mirror.

3.6 Exercise along with Fasting

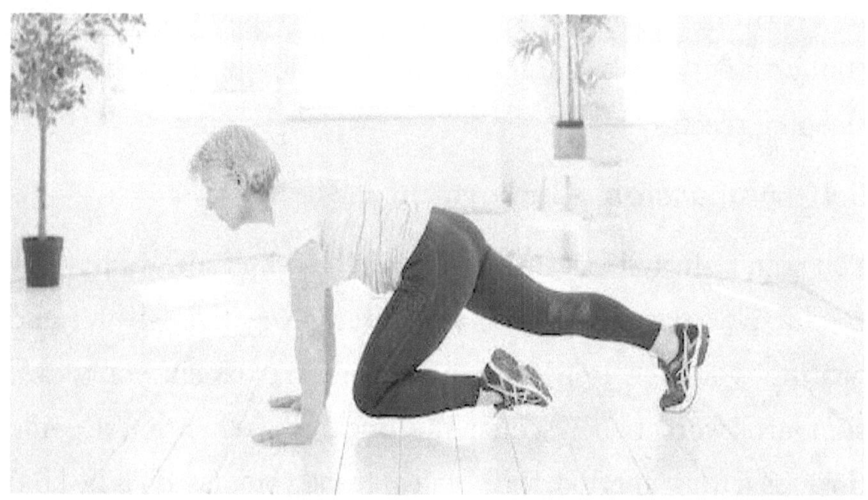

The most prevalent kind of intermittent fasting prevents you from eating in the morning, although this may be your preferred time to exercise. Alternatively, you might exercise in the morning to get the advantages of exercising while fasting. When you're fasting and exercising in the morning, stick to low-impact, low-intensity routines. Fasted workouts include walking, jogging, mild cardio, Pilates, barre, yoga, bodyweight exercises, cycling, and/or a mix of a couple of these. In a fasting condition, do not exercise for more than 60 minutes. If you're new to fasting, you can wake up feeling ravenous (whether you're exercising or not!) It might take anywhere from 10 to 20 days to recover from this, so it's a smart option to exercise in methods that would help you avoid feeling hungry. Don't force yourself to undertake workouts you know you don't like.

Instead, choose things that you know you like since you may discover that you have a greater mind-body connection when you do them on an empty stomach.

Hot flashes, joint discomfort, and sleep issues are some of the signs of menopause that may benefit from physical exercise. Exercise may also help you avoid diabetes, heart disease, and osteoporosis. It also aids in weight loss and the reduction of abdominal fat.

Exercise has such powerful benefits that it affects all physiological systems in your body for the better. Exercises for an Intermittent Fasting Morning Workout:

- Most yoga practitioners prefer to practice on an empty stomach because it gives them a "clean" and "light" sensation that enables them to concentrate only on their breath and body movements.

- Dancing: any type of dance (if you love it) is an enjoyable activity that can help you forget about your hunger. Ballet, barre, Zumba, hip-hop, or any other sort of exercise will suffice.

- Put on your favorite podcast and go for a casual (or not so leisurely) stroll or jog of anywhere from 1-4 kilometers.

- On the treadmill, consider walking at a faster pace (3.5 mph) at an eight inclination or higher than running on a level surface. It's been proven to burn more fat!

- Cycling: fantastic music combined with a terrific ride can make you feel as if you're gliding through the air, whether inside or out.

- Pilates practitioners, like yoga practitioners, seek to be in an empty, "light" state of being.

Intermittent fasting exercise programs to try:

If you only have 30 minutes:

- Take a 15-minute (1-mile) walk outside, or a 1-mile treadmill walks on an incline.

- Spend 15 minutes doing bodyweight workouts such as core exercises, squats, and lunges.

If you only have 45 minutes:

- Take a 20 to 30-minute jog or walk (2 miles) outside, or a 2-mile treadmill walk on an incline.

- Spend 15 minutes doing yoga vinyasas (flowing poses) or 15 minutes doing bodyweight exercises.

If you have one hour:

- Go for some bike ride or a long stroll in the park to see what programs are offered in your region. Invite a buddy to join you for a walk or bike ride or go for a dip on the beach or a pool.

The following items must be included in a comprehensive fitness program:

Aerobic exercise. Try walking, running, swimming, or dancing as a form of exercise. Aerobic exercise strengthens your body's major muscles, which benefits your cardiovascular system as well as your weight. Work your way up to 20 or some more minutes every session, three or four times per week. Make sure that you can pass the "speak test," which requires you to exercise at a rate that allows you to converse.

Strength training is a good thing to do. Lifting hand weights increases your strength & posture, keeps your bones strong, lowers your chance of lower back pain, and tones your muscles. Begin with an eight-repetition hand weight which you can easily carry. Gradually increase the number of repetitions until you can finish 12 in a row.

Stretching. Stretching activities aid in the maintenance of joint flexibility & range of motion. They also help to prevent injuries and muscular discomfort. Yoga & Pilates are excellent stretching exercises that strengthen the core and improve stability.

Remember, all you need to do is move; it doesn't matter what you're doing if it makes you feel good! Make sure you keep hydrated, and if you start to feel weak or dizzy, stop immediately.

3.7 Breaking Your Fast

The 14:10, 16:8, and 18:6 time-restricted eating programs, in which you refrain from meals for 14, 16, and 18 hours each day, respectively, are by far the most common kinds of intermittent fasting. While these sorts of fasts don't need as much preparation as a prolonged fast, there are some fundamental guidelines to follow.

First and foremost, when breaking a fast, stick to whole meals and choose a variety of macronutrients. You don't want a direct blast of carbs (particularly processed carbs) onto an empty stomach. "Definitely avoid carb-dense meals and sugary beverages," adds Amy Shah, M.D., which utilizes IF in her practice. "Moreover, eating a lot of sugar would make fasting the following day much more difficult since your hunger hormones [such as ghrelin] would be elevated."

"A low-glycemic meal of choice might be used to break a fast on a conventional 16:8 schedule," says Ali Miller, R.D., L.D., CDE, a functional medicine practitioner and registered dietitian. "If you are going to eat carbohydrates, make sure you balance them out with protein & fat. Meal number one might be a protein-rich salad, eggs with avocado & vegetables, a home-prepared protein smoothie, or leftover protein with roasted vegetables." When it comes to more rigorous time-restricted eating schedules like 18:6 or 20:4, portion size counts a lot. Even if you're starving when you break your fast, especially if you are new to intermittent fasting, avoid eating a large meal to prevent overloading your digestive system and causing symptoms like bloating. Miller recommends a "hefty snack or light dinner" in most cases. You may integrate the following meals into your 1st post-fast meal by mixing and matching them:

- Foods that have been fermented (pickled veggies, kimchi, sauerkraut, unsweetened kefir)

- Greens with plenty of leaves

- veggies that have been cooked

- Juices from vegetables

- Fruits in their natural state

- Butters made from nuts

- Meats, poultry, eggs, and fish

- Soups and bone broth

- Fats that are good for you (coconut oil, avocado, olive oil, grass-fed butter, & ghee)

-

Longer fasts may be broken in the following ways:

While the "rules" for breaking a smaller, time-restricted fast are rather flexible, how you break a longer fast (that is, a fast of one day or more) requires a little more thought, particularly if you are new to fasting. Not only should you avoid excessive carbohydrates and sugar, but you should also stick to readily digested meals and minimum quantities. "When you're new to Intermittent fasting and stop eating all of a sudden, your body becomes confused and stops generating a lot of digestive fluids," explains Jason Fung, M.D., a fasting specialist & co-author of the new book Life in Fasting Lane. "When you resume eating, your body may lack the necessary nutrients to effectively digest the meal. GI pain and diarrhea are often the outcomes."

The approach is to gradually reintroduce eating. "A healthy soup, as well as some cooked vegetables, may sometimes be a wonderful way of breaking a fast since they are simpler to digest & absorb, Miller concurs, stating, "To lessen digestive & blood sugar stress onto the body, it's ideal for easing off of a fast gradually. I often have people drink bone broth, followed by soft, simple proteins like fish, an hour or two later." Dense foods (think steak) can be too strong right from the beginning, according to Miller, since they demand a lot of digestive enzyme power. If you do consume anything like this, supplement your digestive assistance with digestive herbs or a glass of apple cider vinegar along with your meal. Even if you truly want to, don't stuff yourself upon breaking a prolonged fast. "Portion size does important, particularly if you're fasting for an extended period of time since your stomach isn't used to retaining as much food. When you don't eat as much as you used to, it's as if the stomach contracts. Start with little quantities, see how you react to them, and then go to larger portions if you can tolerate them. Balance what your brain desires with what the body can manage, and stop eating when you're around 75% full. It may be advisable to have many little meals throughout the day on the first day." To regain the energy while breaking a lengthier fast, these meals may be excellent choices:

- Bone broths and nutritious soups are two of my favorite things to eat.

- veggies that have been cooked

- Proteins that are easier to digest, like fish and chicken

Avoid these foods:

As previously stated, excessive carbs, especially refined carbohydrates & sugary drinks, should be avoided when breaking any form of fast to prevent a blood sugar increase. Aside from that, most true whole foods are OK. What you can handle during lengthy fasts may vary (it will rely on the health of your stomach, according to Pedre), and it may take some trial & error to find out what you really can tolerate.

However, specialists advise that you stay away from anything which requires a great deal of digestive work. Raw vegetables, meat, and, on rare occasions, eggs and nuts might be problematic for some individuals to consume shortly after a fast, according to Fung. Also, anything fried or fatty should be avoided until your digestion has been stimulated with milder meals.

Discomfort, bloating, and diarrhea are all possible side effects of consuming these items to break your fast. However, according to Pedre, if you've got a "happy gut" that generates appropriate levels of digestive enzymes, you may break the fast with things like meat and have no problems. It's about the person, so try a few different things to determine what works best for you.

3.8 Tips and Tricks to keep you going

Remember the following principles to make the shift to fasting smoother and to stay on track:

- Shorten your workout, take a break, or drink a glass of water if you feel dizzy or weak while exercising.

- If you've got a bad day when fasting seems too difficult, take a little break and try the following day again.

- Keep yourself hydrated at all times.

- Eat a well-balanced diet that includes protein, healthy fats, fiber, and complex carbohydrates.

- Processed foods should be avoided; you want your meals to help your body instead of empty calories.

- Fast-breakers such as toothpaste (while fasting, use some baking soda paste instead) and drugs with a sugar coating, such as Advil, should be avoided.

- Don't inform your friends, family, or coworkers that you're fasting intermittently until you've established the practice.

- During your fasting intervals, keep yourself engaged and occupied.

- Build up your ideal fasting routine gently if you haven't fasted in quite a long time.

- To avoid hunger and binge eating, eat a lot of veggies in between meals.

- Chewing gum or munching on anything will just make you feel hungrier.

Chapter 4: Misconceptions, Mistakes and FAQs

"A lot of individuals use fasting to lose weight. It has also been demonstrated to increase cognitive function, lower blood sugar, reduce inflammation, improve intestinal health, and make the metabolism more adaptive. However, like with any popular fad, there is a lot of misconception about the eating pattern flying about.

4.1 Common Myths about IF

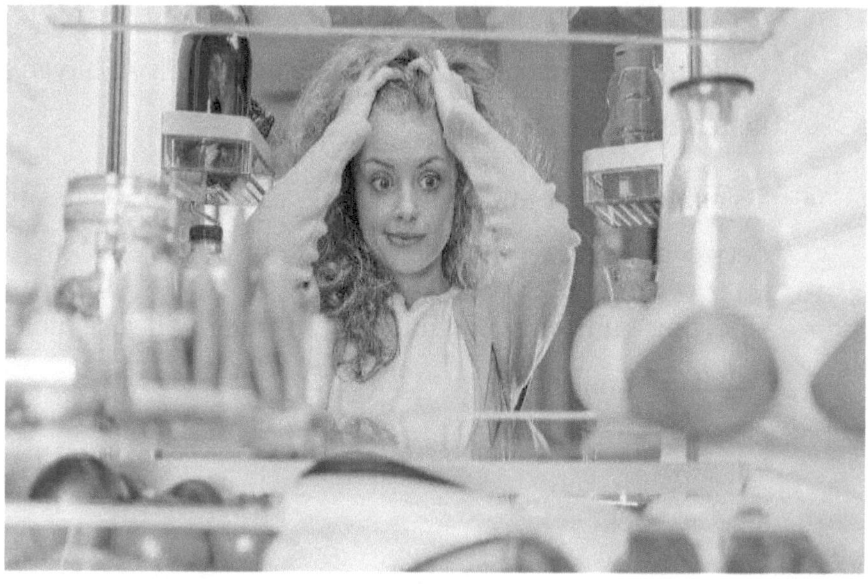

Some dietitians addressed some of the most common fallacies about intermittent fasting to help you separate reality from fantasy.

Myth no.1 Essentially, intermittent fasting is skipping breakfast.

"While this can be true for certain IF adherents," Harbstreet (an IF expert) writes, "this is likely a very simplistic definition." "Those who follow IF, in my experience, plan their meal windows later in the day," she says, "allowing more flexibility for socialising at meals and maybe better aligning with their hunger patterns."

Myth no. 2: IF is a weight-loss magic treatment.

"While intermittent fasting may help with weight reduction, it is not a guarantee," explains Toni Marinucci, a registered dietitian nutritionist in New York & host of the Tips with Toni podcast. "Weight reduction is achieved by achieving a calorie deficit overall, eating less calories than the body burns. As a result, if a person eats more calories than the body burns within their window, they will not lose weight," adds the nutritionist. It's also crucial to remember that "weight is an inconsistent measure of health, and BMI is a eugenicist instrument designed to evaluate weight in certain groups, not individuals," according to Clara Nosek, a registered dietitian nutritionist located in California.

Myth no. 3: IF is the same for everyone.

Intermittent fasting comes in a variety of forms. "Time-restricted eating (TRE) patterns, for example, divide your day between eating and fasting intervals. "The most common version of TRE is known as 16:8, which means you fast for sixteen hrs. and eat all of THE daily calories during an 8-hr. eating window," explains Dr. Gillaspy. "Other typical TRE patterns include daily eating periods ranging from 12 to one hour, a behaviour known OMAD (as 1 meal a day) fasting," she continues. Meanwhile, according to the health coach, "multiple-day feeding patterns that come under the banner of IF include alternative day fasting (ADF) programmes that divide your week between times of eating and fasting, and prolonged fasting schedules which last for 24 hours and more."

Myth no. 4: IF is beneficial to everyone.

Intermittent fasting isn't for everyone, despite its numerous advantages. "Those with a past of an eating problem, as well as those who are presently malnourished or in a fragile or debilitated condition, should avoid fasting." In addition, women who are pregnant or nursing should not start a fasting regimen. Fasting would not be beneficial to children throughout their developing years, according to Dr. Gillaspy. "As a general guideline, if you think about altering your eating or diet habit, you must let your doctor know," the health expert advises.

Myth no. 5: During the eating window, you should eat everything you want.

The feeding window isn't a time to binge on less nutritious foods or compensate for missing eating chances; rather, it is a time to consume a well-balanced meal. A balanced diet is a healthy diet. Whether you follow the IF diet or not, consuming a broad range of nutritious foods such as whole grains, lean meats, healthy fats, fruits, and vegetables is beneficial. After that, if you have a want for anything less nutritional, she suggests allowing for it in moderation.

Myth no. 6: IF might make you lose your mental acuity and concentrate.

"Intermittent fasting has certain unpleasant consequences, such as hunger pains, headaches, or muscular cramps, but mental alertness and attention have not been reported as adverse effects. However, if you begin fasting too soon, you may notice a brief loss of mental acuity and attention. This is why, according to the diet expert, if you are new to fasting, beginning with a 12-hr. fast is the ideal approach to allow the body time to adjust.

Myth no. 7: Intermittent fasting causes your metabolism to slow down.

Fasting, on the other hand, has been demonstrated to raise metabolism and improve adaptability when done for brief periods of time, as in most intermittent fasting regimens like 16:8. Your body's metabolism is the totality of all chemical activities going on within your body." Fasting gives your body the time & rest it needs to produce chemical and hormonal benefits that enhance metabolism. "Fasting increases the levels of some metabolic regulators including norepinephrine and growth hormone. Fasting not only helps your body maintain high levels of metabolically vital hormones, but also it makes you metabolically more flexible, meaning your body can adjust rapidly to the most readily accessible fuel source (carbohydrates or fats).

Myth no. 8: Intermittent fasting causes you to eat too much.

There is a belief that when individuals eat after they break their fast, they would most likely overeat, however data contradicts this. However, it may result in certain disorganized dietary habits. Because of the preoccupation on time, there might be a feeling of urgency when the feeding window 'opens, which could possibly induce someone to consume in a rushed, less attentive fashion."

Myth no. 9 During the fasting time, you should also limit your water consumption.

"Restricting water isn't a smart idea. In fact, you should be conscious of drinking more water since many of you drink water during a meal, and when you aren't eating, you forget that you still have to drink that one glass of water.

Myth no. 10 Your body goes into hunger mode when you fast intermittently.

Although there is no particular caloric threshold or amount of time for your body to reach starvation mode, you can say for sure that it takes more than a day without meals. The 5:2, 16:8 (eating below 600 calories 2 days a week), and 12-hour plans are the most frequent kinds of intermittent fasting, so it's safe to believe that short fasting period won't push your body in starvation mode. If you're thinking of fasting for more than a day, you should assess the risks and advantages and see your doctor before getting started. Long-term fasting has possible advantages, such as weight reduction, greater autophagy, and persistently stable insulin and blood sugar levels, but it also has concerns, such as muscle loss and a decline in metabolism.

4.2 Mistakes to Avoid

Intermittent fasting may be precisely what the doctor prescribed to help you reduce weight and decrease extra body fat. However, before you jump in, you need to learn how to manage a time-restricted diet. Several intermittent fasting blunders might not only sabotage your weight reduction attempts but also put you in danger of gaining weight. Here are the top seven errors to avoid during intermittent fasting:

1. When You Pick the Wrong Fasting Strategy

The kind of intermittent fasting program you choose might lead to the most frequent IF blunder. You've chosen an overly hard fast or the incorrect fasting regimen for you. Consider this: if your body is used to eating every 2 hours, a 24-hour fast would certainly deplete your energy & leave you depressed. Similarly, if your everyday routine keeps you awake late at night, starting your fast at five p.m. is not a good idea. If you begin your fast early in the evening, you risk staying up later than planned without eating.

2. When you complete a fast, you eat too much.

It's no secret that finishing your first fast will make you feel tremendously accomplished. This pride, however, should not be used as an excuse to overindulge. After a fast, you'll most likely be hungry. And you could believe that the calories you ate after you broke your fast would compensate for the calories you lost while fasting. If you're feeling this way, it's possible that it'll rationalize your want to binge and undo all of your hard work. One of the main advantages of IF is that it lowers insulin levels and encourages your body to use alternate sources of energy to burn fat. When you eat after you've broken your fast, your levels of blood sugar & insulin levels jump quickly, ruining your effort and leaving you with a nagging headache, nausea, and shakiness.

3. You Don't Eat Enough before Starting a Fast

The eating time leading up to your fast is referred to as your "feasting window" for a reason: you're intended to eat until you're satisfied. Ghrelin, the hunger hormone, urges the brain to eat when you're hungry. When you limit eating, your ghrelin levels rise, intensifying your hunger. During a fast, high amounts of this hormone might make you feel hungry and depleted of energy.

4. You Indulge in Unhealthy Eating During Your Feasting Period

Aside from not having enough during your feasting window, overeating or consuming unhealthy meals before or after the fast is another typical intermittent fasting error. Though your body benefits the most when fasting, the meals you eat after or before the fast are what will re-energize you for your next fast. So, if you load up on meals that temporarily raise your sugar level or make you feel full, you won't get the full advantages of a fast. The success of the fast is mostly determined by what you consume while you're not fasting.

5. You Are Not Consuming Enough Water

Another typical intermittent fasting blunder is to consume caffeinated tea or coffee first thing in the morning instead of water. Just from the moisture in your breath, you lost roughly a liter of water while sleeping. Caffeinated beverages have a diuretic effect, which makes you want to pee more often, dehydrating your body even more. Furthermore, a large quantity of caffeine may have a detrimental effect on blood sugar levels, making you extra insulin resistant & more prone to accumulate fat.

6. You lead a sedentary lifestyle.

Your lifestyle choices have a big influence on how well you lose weight. Your weight loss is greatly influenced by the foods you consume, the quantity of sleep you receive, and even your stress levels. Similarly, if you don't exercise or stay active throughout your fast, your results may stall. If you want to grow muscle and sculpt your ideal body, intermittent fasting, exercise, & an active lifestyle are important.

7. When your results aren't immediate, you give up.

When you don't experience instant effects from intermittent fasting, you make the mistake of giving up. Realistically, losing weight and shedding stubborn body fat will take time. After your first weight reduction, you'll bloat quickly or shed water weight and lose 1-2 pounds each week. Don't be disheartened if you don't lose weight soon; studies suggest that if you lose weight too rapidly, it's more likely to return.

4.3 FAQs

Intermittent fasting is more accurately described as an eating pattern than a diet in the traditional sense. These are the most common intermittent fasting questions.

1. Isn't it true that you should eat every three hours? How is it, therefore, that such extended intervals between meals are healthy?

When it refers to weight reduction or calorie burning, eating multiple little meals during the day may not be enough. You'll wind up in the same location whether you eat the same number of calories in ten meals or 1 meal. In fact, even when the overall amount of calories daily is the same, a few studies have indicated that eating two big meals per day promotes insulin sensitivity & promotes weight reduction in certain people better than eating frequent little meals.

2. Is it possible to exercise while fasting?

Of course, yes. Not only does nutrition have a role in weight reduction, but so does exercise. During it is feasible to exercise whilst fasting, care is advised. Your body's glycogen reserves are depleted when you fast. As a result, when you exercise, your body begins burning the fat for energy that helps you lose weight. You should organize your training sessions and schedules intelligently around those fueled and empty time intervals for the best outcomes. So, perform your cardio before or after your weight lifting workouts, and lift during or after the meal windows.

3. Is it permissible to consume any liquids?

It all depends on the beverage you're drinking and the sort of IF diet you're on. When fasting, a good rule of thumb is to limit any calorie liquids. You may have a cup of black coffee or a cup of black tea (no sugar). Water is a naturally calorie-free beverage, so there is no need to limit yourself. Additionally, water may be essential while fasting for proper hydration, as well as to fill your stomach and satisfy hunger. To offer some diversity, fruit-infused water might be utilized. Not to mention, avoid soda and alcoholic beverages.

4. Is it true that intermittent fasting causes muscle loss?

When you lose weight, both fat & muscle mass are often lost. If your body starts a calorie deficit, it's more probable that you will lose muscle mass as well as lose weight when fasting. As a result, the solution is simple. Count the calories and make sure you're eating enough to maintain your weight. Inactivity or not utilizing muscle is also a major source of muscle loss than IF, according to research. So keep working out or doing resistance training to help keep your muscles strong.

5. Is there anybody who shouldn't fast?

Intermittent fasting should be avoided by pregnant women, nursing women, and diabetics. Furthermore, those with eating disorders such as anorexia or bulimia nervosa should not fast intermittently. Also, persons who participate in difficult sports, endurance, and strength training exercises rely on optimal nutritional timings, which might be thrown off by this diet plan.

6. Skipping meals causes your body to go into hunger mode, slowing your metabolism since it thinks it's a "period of famine." Is this correct?

IF is a great way to lose weight. Fasting for a brief amount of time may actually help your metabolism & metabolic health, rather than slowing it down.

7. Can a person eat as much as he wants during the eating window since he'll be missing a meal and compensating for it anyway?

Intermittent fasting focuses on "when you eat" rather than "what you eat." Intermittent fasting does, in fact, provide you greater flexibility to eat anything you want. However, some individuals make the mistake of consuming too much processed & junk food in the feeding window, negating all of the fasting advantages. If you want to be healthy in general, cut down on refined sugars and replace junk and processed foods with more plant-based foods.

8. Will a person feel hungry and exhausted for the rest of the day since he is starving himself?

Yes, you may feel weary and sluggish at first, particularly if you're new to intermittent fasting. Your body has a lower energy level than normal. Fasting also raises stress levels and might affect your mental state & sleep schedule. However, As you grow more used to intermittent fasting, it becomes simpler. When your body adapts to its new power consumption pattern, this affects the way it functions, including hunger symptoms.

9. What's the most effective method of using IF for weight loss?

The 5:2 diet is a way of eating that encourages you to eat less this diet requires you to eat regularly five days a week and limit your calorie consumption to 500-600 calories two days a week. You may then go to 14-hour fasting and ultimately escalate to 16-hour fasting.

10. Is it necessary to give up the social life during intermittent fasting?

You may not have to forego those late-night meals, birthday celebrations, or lunches with family & friends. Meal preparation and execution will assist you in resolving issues with eating outdoors. You may adjust your plan to fit a social engagement if one arises. You may also take a rest from intermittent fasting every now and then and restart your fasting routine after a weekend trip, a vacation, or even an evening out with friends if necessary.

11. What are your thoughts on intermittent fasting?

You've all probably fasted at some time in your lives owing to a variety of religious reasons. Have you ever considered the scientific basis behind it? To determine for yourself whether intermittent fasting is healthy for you, you must first comprehend the idea and its impact on your biological systems. This diet, however, may be quite effective for weight reduction if followed properly with healthy food alternatives and appropriate activity.

12. The disadvantages or problems that may occur as a result of intermittent fasting?

You may get ravenously hungry as a result of your fasting, making you inefficient at work. It may make you feel tired and nauseated and lower your blood sugar levels. Intermittent fasting may be detrimental to mindful eating. In women, it may lead to digestive problems, dietary deficits, electrolyte irregularities, and fertility & reproductive disorders. As a result, it's always a good idea to speak with a dietitian who can provide you with recommendations depending on your metabolism and overall health.

4.4   Tasty   Food   Choices   Without Compromising IF Results

If you've been researching IF for a while, you must have come across the many fasting recipes for bakes, puddings, and cakes that, although comfortingly low in calories, are heavy in processed & refined ingredients and poor in nutrients. If you want to stay healthy for the rest of your life, avoid these foods. Fasting may be beneficial if you choose the appropriate foods and ingredients, as well as recipes which not only taste great but also set you on the road to better health and life. Plus, you'll be able to reach the right number on your bathroom scales. There are a few things to bear in mind:

- You won't have to drink huge quantities of water and peck at birdseed or subsist on low-calorie junk food if you include whole foods in your fasting days. Instead, you will be capable of eating properly and abundantly in a natural way. You'll also satisfy your nutritional requirements on fasting days and get the most nutrients out of each meal. Welcome to a reasonable, straightforward, and long-term approach to IF, with balanced meals created with nutrient-dense, unprocessed whole foods to help you feel more energized.

- Whole foods often have fewer calories & more nutrients than the other foods, allowing you to load more on your plate while still sticking to a low-calorie, low-fat diet. Intermittent fasting has been shown to improve health, lifespan, and weight reduction over time. It entails limiting calorie consumption to about 2090 kJ (500kcal) for women & 2510 kJ (600kcal) for males on a regular basis (say, two days per week).

- An intermittent fasting regimen for women that incorporates high-quality saturated fats from foods like eggs, coconut oil, and grass-fed butter is critical for signaling to their bodies that they are in a safe environment for hormone production. Traditional fasting may cause brain fog, tiredness, anger, and chilly hands. Therefore this will help. These items are very crucial to incorporate to prevent any unwanted disordered eating behaviors that may result from calorie restriction & fat avoidance.

- Fats would be included in a safe fasting strategy for women at all times. Poached eggs with spinach and avocado for breakfast, a mid-day smoothie with coconut water, & a vegetable & bone broth soup with a tiny quantity of coconut oil or ghee for supper is a lovely, mild intermittent fasting choice that will promote hormone function while supporting weight reduction and detoxifying. In addition, adding Himalayan salt or Celtic sea salt to filtered water and meals works wonderfully.

Intermittent fasting for women that is hormone-friendly:

1) Use herb-filled frittatas or omelets instead of pastry-bound quiches or flans. You get the same flavor punch without the carb-heavy pastry.

2) For a lower sugar intake, use frozen or fresh berries for watermelon & other high-fructose fruits.

3) Use vegetarian pasta instead of ordinary spaghetti. Make "zoodles" or "coodles" using zucchini or cucumber, then serve raw or steamed. Using a spiralizer, vegetable peeler, or mandolin, make thin ribbons.

4) Use cauliflower "rice" instead of rice. Just shred cauliflower and pan-fry or steam it with lime juice or lemon. For a splash of color, add a little turmeric.

5) Swap the bread and wrappers with lettuce leaves, steaming bok Choy, cabbage, or seaweed wraps.

Chapter 5: Tasty, Easy and Quick Recipes

Breakfast Recipes

1. Buddha Breakfast Bowl

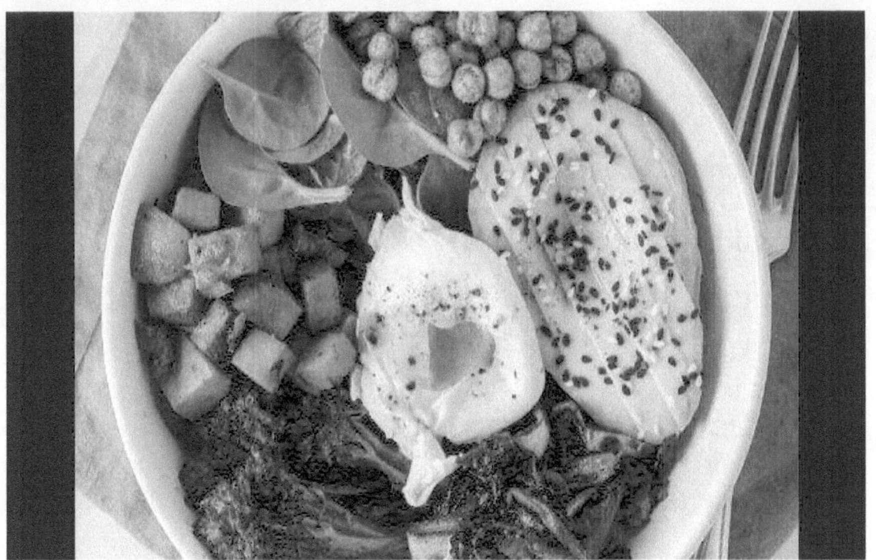

Ready in: 25 mins.

Serves: 2

Difficulty: easy

Ingredients:

- 2 precooked Paleo sausages

- 2 eggs (pastured), poached

- 1 cup of cauliflower rice

- 1 sliced avocado

- Grass-fed ghee to cook

- 1/4 sliced cucumber

- Garnishing: sliced chili, fresh herbs, spring onions (sliced), a lemon wedge, salt to taste

- 2 handfuls of leafy greens (organic), lightly steamed

Directions:

- Preheat a frying pan on medium.

- Add 1-2 tablespoons of ghee and let it melt all through the pan. Cook until the cauliflower rice is done to your liking.

- Place leafy greens on a platter or in a big mixing bowl.

- Place the cauliflower rice with the leafy leaves once it's ready.

- Reheat the sausages in the same frying pan.

- Meanwhile, arrange the avocado, cucumber slices, & poached eggs on the top of cauliflower rice & leafy greens as desired.

- When sausages are done, add them to the bowl with the remaining ingredients.

- Garnish with preferred garnishes, then serve & enjoy!

Nutritional values per serving:

Total Calories: 484kcal, **Fats:** 40g, **Carbohydrates:** 13g, **Protein:** 25g

2. Garlic Spinach & Smoked Salmon Breakfast Sandwich

Ready in: 25 mins.

Serves: 2-4

Difficulty: easy

Ingredients:

- 8 slices of a sandwich vessel, any preferred
- 4 tbsp. of coconut oil
- 4 oz. of smoked salmon
- 4 tbsp. of powdered eggs (organic) or 2 whole eggs (pasture-raised),
- 9 oz. of fresh spinach
- 4 tbsp. of water
- 1/2 lemon
- 2 cloves of garlic or 1/2 tsp. of garlic powder

Directions:

- If you're using powdered eggs, be sure to rehydrate them in water first. Allow settling for 5 minutes after stirring.

- In the meanwhile, heat the burner to medium. Put 2 tbsp. Coconut oil in a pan. Both sides of the sandwich bread should be toasted. Mince the cloves of garlic while the bread is browning.

- Add the remaining 2 tbsp. Coconut oil in the pan after all of the slices have been roasted. Garlic should be cooked for 1-2 minutes. Cook for 2-3 minutes or until spinach has wilted.

- Toss in the eggs. Stir carefully to scramble the eggs and cook for 2-3 minutes or until set. Add a splash of lemon to the finish.

- On toast, layer the smoked salmon & garlic spinach scramble. Eat!

Nutritional values per serving:

Total Calories: 304.7kcal, **Fats:** 9.2g, **Carbohydrates:** 39.8g, **Protein:** 17.5g

3. Collagen Cookies

Ready in: 35 mins.

Serves: 12

Difficulty: easy

Ingredients:

- ½ cup of almond flour
- 2 eggs
- ½ cup of shredded coconut
- ½ cup of pecans
- ½ cup of sliced almonds
- ½ cup of pumpkin seeds
- 1/3 cup of roasted almond butter
- ½ cup of chocolate chips, sugar-free
- 1/3 cup of monk fruit-erythritol granulated blend
- 2 and ½ tbsp. of Bulletproof Collagen Protein (Vanilla)
- 2 tbsp. of ground flax meal
- 2-3 tsp. of cinnamon
- 1 tsp. of vanilla extract
- 2-3 tsp. of ginger powder

Directions:

- Preheat the oven up to 350 degrees Fahrenheit.
- Line two baking pans with parchment paper.

- In a mixing dish, combine all cookie ingredients.

- Roll the dough into balls using your hands oiled with coconut oil. Place the cookies on the prepped baking pans and press them flat and even.

- Bake the tray for 20-25 mins, or till golden & cooked through.

- Remove the cookies from the oven & set them aside to rest.

- For a keto-friendly breakfast, serve with a cup of Bulletproof Coffee.

Nutritional values per serving:

Total Calories: 289kcal, **Fats:** 21g, **Carbohydrates:** 17g, **Protein:** 8g

---

4. Breakfast Pizza

Ready in: 25 mins.

Serves: 2

Difficulty: easy

Ingredients:

- 2 tbsp. of coconut flour

- 2 cups of grated cauliflower

- 1/2 tsp. of salt

- 1 tbsp. of Psyllium husk powder

- 4 eggs

- Toppings: avocado, smoked salmon, herbs, olive oil, spinach

Directions:

- Preheat the oven up to 350 degrees Fahrenheit. Use parchment paper to line a sheet pan or a pizza tray.

- Blend all ingredients (excluding toppings) in a mixing bowl and stir to combine. Allow Psyllium husk and coconut flour to absorb liquid & thicken for 5 minutes before serving.

- Pour the morning pizza foundation into the pan with care. Form it into a circular, even pizza crust using your hands.

- Bake for 10-15 minutes, or until thoroughly cooked and golden brown.

- Remove the morning pizza from the oven & top with your preferred toppings. Warm the dish before serving.

Nutritional values per serving:

Total Calories: 454kcal, **Fats:** 31g, **Carbohydrates:** 26g, **Protein:** 22g

5. Matcha Berry Smoothie

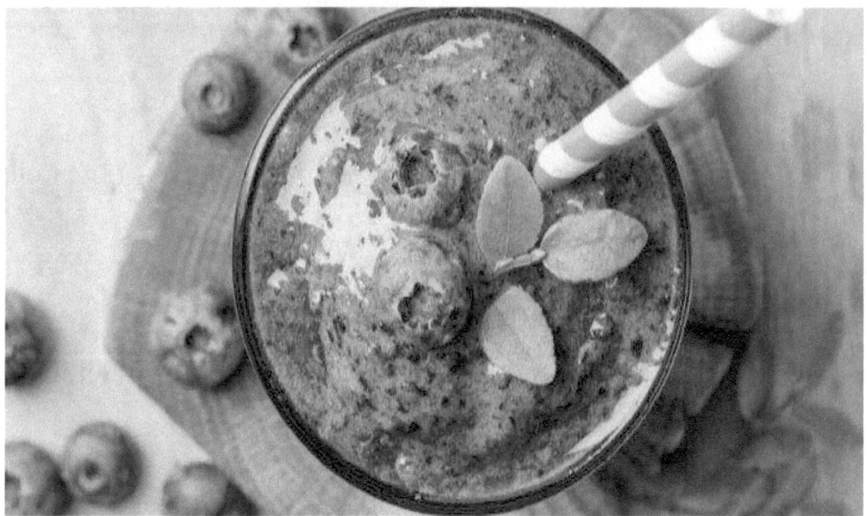

Ready in: 5 mins.

Serves: 2

Difficulty: easy

Ingredients:

- 1 cup of filtered water

- 1 cup of coconut milk

- 1-1.5 cups of frozen organic berries

- 1 tbsp. of Oil

- 1/2 avocado

- 1 scoop of Vanilla Bean Collagen Energy Protein

- 1 tsp. of matcha powder

- 1 scoop of Bulletproof Inner-Fuel Prebiotic

- 1/2-1 tsp. of vanilla extract

- Optional: Ice & sweetener of choice, according to taste

Directions:

- In a blender, combine all of the ingredients and mix until totally smooth.

- Taste and make any necessary adjustments.

- Pour into 2 glasses and serve right away.

Nutritional values per serving:

Total Calories: 496kcal, **Fats:** 40.9g, **Carbohydrates:** 30g, **Protein:** 10.7g

6. Coconut Flour Breakfast Pancakes

Ready in: 15 mins.

Serves: 3

Difficulty: easy

Ingredients:

- 1/2 tsp. of baking soda

- 1/2 cup of coconut flour (50g)

- 2 tbsp. of coconut oil, melted

- 1 tsp. of vanilla

- 4 organic eggs (pasture-raised), room temperature

- 1/2 tsp. of Ceylon cinnamon

- 1/2 cup of almond milk, unsweetened

- 1/2 cup of coconut cream (the unsweetened and thick part of the canned coconut cream)

- Coconut oil or Grass-fed Ghee for cooking

- 1/4 tsp. of Himalayan salt

Directions:

- Add all the ingredients except ghee to a high-powered blender and mix until smooth, scraping down the sides as required.

- Add sufficient ghee to cover the bottom of a medium pan over medium heat. Pour roughly 1/2 cup batter onto the skillet after it has heated up. Cook until golden brown on 1 side, then turn and cook until golden brown on the other side. Set aside & continue to fry until there is no more batter.

- Hot coconut flour pancakes with grass-fed ghee, fruit, or other keto-friendly toppings

Nutritional values per serving:

Total Calories: 244kcal, **Fats:** 23g, **Carbohydrates:** 4.9g, **Protein:** 5.5g

7. Perfect Basic Hard Boiled Eggs

Ready in: 21 mins.

Serves: 6

Difficulty: easy

Ingredients:

- Some water, as required

- 6 eggs (large)

Directions:

- In a medium saucepan, crack the eggs. Cover it with water 1 inch above the eggs. Place high heat on the stovetop.

- Bring the water to a boil. Remove from heat & cover immediately. Allow for 18-20 minutes of resting time.

- Holding the pan on a slant, pour tap water into the saucepan, enabling the hot water to escape. Allow eggs to rest in the cold water for 1 to 2 minutes before peeling.

Nutritional values per serving:

Total Calories: 71.5kcal, **Fats:** 42g, **Carbohydrates:** 0.4g, **Protein:** 6.3g

8. Peach Smoothie

Ready in: 5 mins.

Serves: 1

Difficulty: easy

Ingredients:

- ¼ cup of coconut milk (adjust for a thinner or thicker smoothie)

- 1 cup of frozen peaches

- ½ tsp. of almond flavoring

- ½ cup of Greek yogurt

Directions:

- In a high-powered blender, combine peaches and almond flavoring.

- Check the thickness and make any necessary adjustments. If you want it thinner, add more milk, and if you want it thicker, add more peaches.

- Berries, Chia seeds, and slivered almonds are lovely additions.

- Enjoy.

Nutritional values per serving:

Total Calories: 351.3kcal, **Fats:** 111g, **Carbohydrates:** 61.6g, **Protein:** 2.7g

9. Avocado & Poached Eggs Toast

Ready in: 15 mins.

Serves: 4

Difficulty: easy

Ingredients:

- 2 avocados (ripe)

- 4 eggs

- 2 tsp. of lemon juice

- 1 cup of cheese (edam, grated, gruyere or any other)

- 4 slices of thick bread

- 4 tsp. of butter (for spreading it on toast)

- salt & black pepper (freshly ground)

Directions:

- Use your preferred way to poach eggs.

- Meanwhile, remove the stones from the avocados and cut them in half.

- Scoop the flesh in a bowl with a spoon, then add the lemon juice, salt, and pepper.

- Using a fork, mash the potatoes roughly.

- Butter the toast and smear it with butter.

- Top each piece of buttered bread with the avocado mixture and a poached egg.

- Serve immediately with a sprinkle of grated cheese.

- With grilled or fresh tomato halves on the side, they are very delicious.

Nutritional values per serving:

Total Calories: 439.8kcal, **Fats:** 280g, **Carbohydrates:** 26.6g, **Protein:** 16.2g

10. French Almond Vanilla Granola

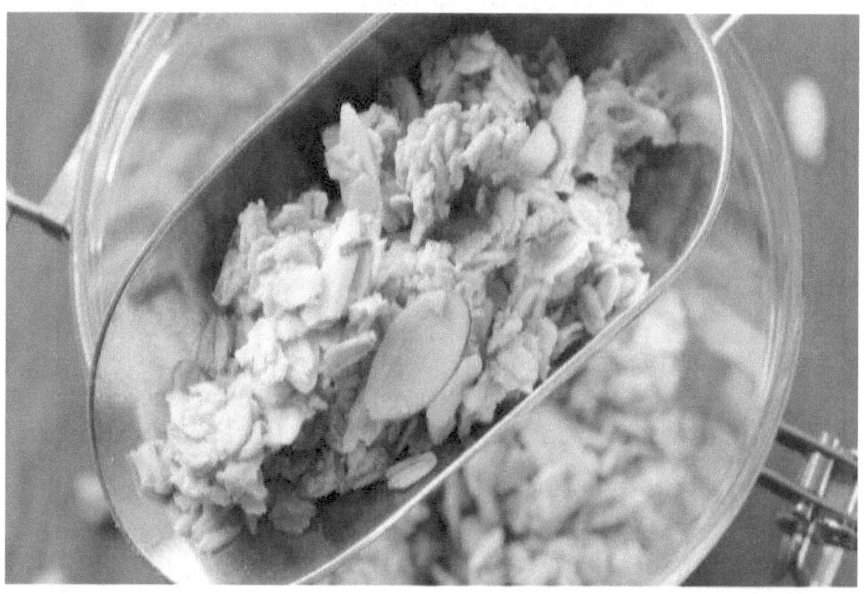

Ready in: 1 hr. 10 mins.

Serves: 12

Difficulty: easy

Ingredients:

- ½ cup of sliced almonds

- 3 ½ cups of old fashioned oats

- ½ cup of water

- ¼ tsp. of salt

- ½ cup of natural cane sugar

- 1 tbsp. of vanilla extract

- ¼ cup of organic canola oil or Grapeseed oil

Directions:

- Preheat oven up to 200 degrees F. With parchment paper, coat a rimmed, large cookie sheet.

- Mix the oats & almonds in a big mixing bowl.

- Stir the salt and sugar into the water in a small saucepan on medium heat. Cook, stirring constantly until the sugar has dissolved. Remove the pan from the heat. Combine the canola oil & vanilla extract in a mixing bowl. Stir in the oat & almond mixture until everything is well mixed.

- Bake for two hours, or until mixture is dry to the touch, on a prepared baking sheet. Stirring is not allowed! Remove from the oven & set aside to cool before slicing into bits. Keep the container airtight.

Nutritional values per serving:

Total Calories: 187.1kcal, **Fats:** 71g, **Carbohydrates:** 25.3g, **Protein:** 3.9g

Lunch Recipes

1. Avocado Quesadillas

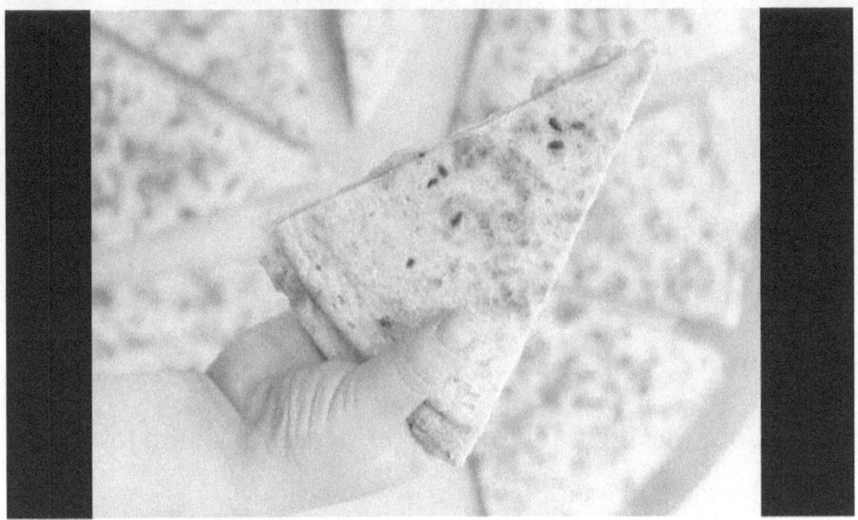

Ready in: 31 mins.

Serves: 2

Difficulty: easy

Ingredients:

- 1 avocado (ripe), pitted, peeled and chopped into 1/4 inch pieces

- 2 tomatoes (vine-ripe), seeded & chopped into 1/4 inch pieces

- 1 tbsp. of chopped red onion

- 1/4 tsp. of Tabasco sauce

- 2 tsp. of fresh lemon juice

- salt and black pepper

- 3 tbsp. of fresh coriander, chopped

- 1/4 cup of sour cream

- 24 inches of flour tortillas

- 1 1/3 cups of Monterey Jack cheese, shredded

- 1/2 tsp. of vegetable oil

Directions:

- Combine the tomatoes, onion, avocado, lemon juice, and Tabasco in a small bowl.

- Season with salt & pepper to taste.

- Mix sour cream, salt, coriander, and pepper to taste in a separate small bowl.

- Brush the tops of the tortillas with oil and place them on a baking pan.

- 2-4 inches from the flame, broil tortillas until lightly golden.

- Sprinkle cheese evenly over tortillas and broil until melted.

- To create 2 quesadillas, spread the avocado mixture equally over 2 tortillas & top each with 1 of the remaining tortillas and cheese side down.

- Cut the quesadillas into four wedges on a chopping board.

- Serve heated with a spoonful of the sour cream mixture on top of each slice.

Nutritional values per serving:

Total Calories: 794kcal, **Fats:** 460g, **Carbohydrates:** 58.7g, **Protein:** 29.2 g

---

2. Cheesy Veggie Packed Chicken Salad

Ready in: 35 mins.

Serves: 1-2

Difficulty: easy

Ingredients:

- 1/4 cup of celery, finely chopped

- 1 cup of cooked skinless, boneless chicken breast, cubed

- 1/4 cup of carrot, shaved in ribbons

- 2 1/2 tbsp. of fat-free mayonnaise

- 1/2 cup of roughly chopped Baby Spinach

- 2 tbsp. of sour cream, nonfat

- 2 tsp. of Dijon mustard

- 1/8 tsp. of dried parsley

- 1/4 cup of sharp cheddar cheese (reduced-fat), shredded

Directions:

- In a mixing dish, combine all ingredients and coat well with the mayonnaise mixture.

- Refrigerate for 30 minutes at least, but it's better if you do it one night before.

- Serve.

Nutritional values per serving:

Total Calories: 364.5kcal, **Fats:** 81g, **Carbohydrates:** 15.3g, **Protein:** 53.2g

---

3. Fried Vegan 'Fish' Tacos

Ready in: 50 mins.

Serves: 8 small

Difficulty: medium

Ingredients:

- 2 cups of panko breadcrumbs

- 14 ounces of silken tofu

- 1/2 cup of plain flour

- 1 tsp. of smoked paprika

- ½ tsp. of salt

- ½ tsp. of cayenne pepper

- ½ cup of non-dairy milk

- 1 tsp. of ground cumin

- vegetable oil to fry

- 1 avocado, ripe

- ¼ head of cabbage, finely shredded

- vegan mayonnaise for serving

- 8 tortillas (small)

For Pickled Onion:

- ¼ cup of apple cider vinegar

- 1 peeled red onion, finely sliced

- 1 tsp. of salt

- 1 tbsp. of sugar

Directions:

- To remove excess moisture, pat the tofu with a few pieces of kitchen paper. Break the tofu into roughly 1-inch pieces with a knife

- In a large shallow dish, combine the breadcrumbs.

- In a separate large shallow bowl, combine the flour, smoked paprika, salt, cayenne, and cumin.

- In a third broad shallow dish, pour the milk.

- Toss the tofu pieces in the flour, then the milk, then the breadcrumbs, and place them on a baking sheet.

- Fill the deep frying pan with vegetable oil to a depth of 1/2 inch. Place on medium heat & let the oil heat up. If a breadcrumb begins to bubble & brown, the oil is ready. Fry pieces of breaded tofu till golden beneath, then flip and finish cooking until golden all over. To drain, place on a baking sheet that is lined with kitchen paper. Rep with the rest of the tofu.

- To make the pickled onion, combine the following ingredients in a small bowl.

- In a small saucepan, heat the salt, apple cider vinegar, and sugar until steaming. Pour the boiling vinegar over the thinly chopped red onion into a dish or jar. Allow it to soften and become pink for 30 minutes at least.

- Serve hot fried tofu with pickled onion, avocado, vegan mayo, and shredded cabbage in warmed tortillas.

Nutritional values per serving:

Total Calories: 378.3kcal, **Fats:** 97g, **Carbohydrates:** 58.2g, **Protein:** 12.2g

---

4. Chicken Breasts & Avocado Tapenade

Ready in: 15 mins.

Serves: 4

Difficulty: easy

Ingredients:

- 1 tbsp. of grated lemon peel
- 4 skinless, boneless chicken breast halves
- 5 tbsp. of lemon juice (fresh), divided
- 1 tsp. of olive oil, divided
- 2 tbsp. of olive oil, divided
- 1 clove of garlic, finely chopped
- 1/4 tsp. of ground black pepper
- 1/2 tsp. of salt
- 2 cloves of garlic, roasted & mashed
- 1/4 tsp. of fresh ground pepper
- 1/2 tsp. of sea salt
- 1 tomato (medium), seeded & finely chopped

- 3 tbsp. of capers, rinsed

- ¼ cup of green pimento olive, stuffed (small), thinly sliced

- 1 Hass avocado (large), ripe and finely chopped

- 2 tbsp. of basil leaves (fresh), finely sliced

Directions:

- Combine chicken, lemon peel, and 2 tbsp. Lemon juice, 2 tbsp. Oil, garlic, salt, and pepper in a sealable plastic bag. Refrigerate for 30 mins after sealing the bag.

- Combine the remaining 3 tbsp. Lemon juice, 1/2 teaspoon olive oil, roasted garlic, sea salt, and freshly ground pepper in a mixing bowl. Set aside the tomato, capers, green olives, basil, and avocado.

- Remove the chicken from the bag and toss out the marinade. Grill for 4 to 5 minutes on each side over medium-hot coals or until the desired level of doneness is reached.

- Avocado Tapenade is a great addition to this dish.

Nutritional values per serving:

Total Calories: 277.1kcal, **Fats:** 147g, **Carbohydrates:** 6.9g, **Protein:** 26.4g

5. Lamb Tacos & Cauliflower Tortillas

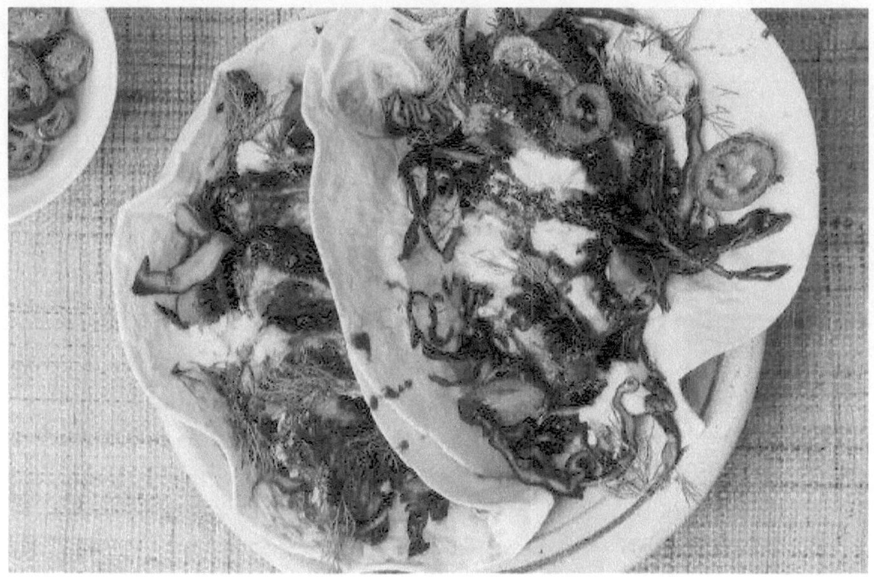

Ready in: 3 hr. 25 mins.

Serves: 6

Difficulty: easy

Ingredients:

Lamb Shoulder (Slow-Cooked):

- 2 cups of pastured chicken stock

- 1.5 pounds of lamb shoulder

- 1 tbsp. of avocado oil

- 1 tbsp. of chopped parsley

- 3 sprigs rosemary

- 2 cloves of garlic, minced

- 1 tsp. of cumin

- 1 tbsp. of Bulletproof Grass-Fed Ghee

- Salt & pepper to taste

Cauliflower Tortillas:

- 1 egg (large)

- 1 cup of cauliflower rice (cooked & cooled)

- 1 tsp. of avocado oil

- ½ tbsp. of Psyllium husk powder

- 1 tbsp. of almond flour

- ½ tsp. of xanthan gum

- ½ tsp. of onion powder

- ½ tsp. of parsley leaves (dried)

- ½ tsp. of garlic powder

- ½ tsp. of cracked black pepper

- ½ tsp. of salt

- 1 tsp. of cilantro (fresh), finely chopped

- 1 sliced radish

Directions:

Lamb Marinade:

- Small incisions should be cut through the lamb's shoulder. Freshly chopped parsley, 1 tbsp. Avocado oil, cumin, minced garlic, and salt & pepper are slathered over the top. Marinate for 6-12 hrs. or overnight in the refrigerator.

Lamb Shoulder:

- Preheat the oven up to 275 degrees Fahrenheit. Preheat a medium-high burner with a Dutch oven. Ghee should be melted, and lamb shoulder should be seared on both sides.

- Bring the braising liquid to a boil with the chicken stock. Scatter rosemary sprigs on top.

- Cover the Dutch oven and transfer it to the oven from the burner. Allow 3 hours to braise.

- Remove the lamb shoulder from the oven and set it aside to rest while the cauliflower tortillas bake.

Cauliflower Tortillas:

- Preheat the oven up to 375 degrees Fahrenheit.

- Wring cooked & cooled cauliflower rice with cheesecloth in stages until no liquid remains.

- Combine the cauliflower rice, egg, and additional ingredients in a mixing bowl. Using a spatula or clean hands, thoroughly combine the ingredients.

- Once a tacky dough has formed, divide it into six balls and set them on 1-2 oiled and parchment-lined baking sheets.

- Smooth dough balls with the back of a spoon until 6 tortillas forms form.

- Bake the cauliflower tortillas for 18-20 minutes, turning halfway during the baking time.

- Allow 5-6 minutes for the tortillas to cool once they've been cooked.

Assembly of Tacos:

- Pull soft lamb shoulder flesh apart with a fork.

- Top the cauliflower tortilla with a hefty tablespoon of pulled lamb shoulder. Serve with sliced radish & chopped cilantro on top. Repeat until all 6 tacos have been prepared.

- Enjoy your guilt-free keto lamb tacos!

Nutritional values per serving:

Total Calories: 203kcal, **Fats:** 11g, **Carbohydrates:** 6g, **Protein:** 18g

6. Thai Grilled Steak with Low-Carb Salad

Ready in: 40 mins.

Serves: 2

Difficulty: medium

Ingredients:

- 1 bok Choy head, lengthwise sliced into quarters

- 1 tbsp. of grass-fed ghee or coconut oil

- 1/4 red cabbage (medium), roughly shredded

- Two hanger steaks or top sirloin (4-ounce) about thickness 3/4-inch

- 1 carrot (medium), spiralized

- Optional: Fresh cilantro, fresh lime juice, sliced radishes, or chopped green onions for garnishing

Marinade Ingredients:

- 1/2 tbsp. of ground ginger

- 2 tbsp. of coconut aminos

- 1/2 coriander (ground)

- 1/2 tbsp. of fresh lime juice

- 1 tsp. of raw honey

- 1/2 tsp. of salt

Directions:

- Whisk together the marinade ingredients in a mixing basin. Toss the steaks in the basin with the marinade. Cover and set aside for 20 minutes to marinate. (If you want to marinate the steaks for longer, put them in the fridge.)

- Bring 1 inch of water to a boil in a pan along with a steamer basket. Reduce to low heat and steam the bok Choy for approximately 6 minutes, or till tender. Remove the item and place it away.

- Sauté the red cabbage in coconut oil in a skillet over medium heat until soft. Remove the cabbage and add the carrots into the pan, cooking for another 2-3 minutes.

- Warm a cast-iron pan over medium-high heat. Add the steaks & cook for 2-3 minutes once the pan is hot. Cook for another 2 minutes after flipping the steaks.

- Allow the steaks to rest for 3-5 minutes before slicing against the grain.

- Assemble the Thai salad by arranging the veggies and adding the meat on top. If desired, add garnishes.

Nutritional values per serving:

Total Calories: 438kcal, **Fats:** 24g, **Carbohydrates:** 20.8g, **Protein:** 30g

7. Lentil Burgers

Ready in: 1 hr. 10 mins.

Serves: 8-10

Difficulty: medium

Ingredients:

- 2 and ½ cups of water

- 1 cup of well-rinsed dried lentils

- ½ tsp. of salt

- ½ onion (medium), diced

- 1 tbsp. of olive oil

- 1 diced carrot

- 1 tbsp. of soy sauce

- 1 tsp. of pepper

- ¾ cup of breadcrumbs

- ¾ cup of finely ground rolled oats

Directions:

- Lentils should be cooked for 45 minutes in salted water. The lentils will be mushy & most of the liquid will have evaporated.

- In a little amount of oil, fry the onions & carrots until tender, approximately 5 minutes.

- Combine the cooked ingredients, pepper, oats, soy sauce, and bread crumbs, in a mixing bowl.

- Form the batter into patties while it is still heated; it will create 8-10 burgers.

- After that, the burgers may be baked for 15 minutes at 200°C or shallow fried for one to two mins on each side.

Nutritional values per serving:

Total Calories: 176.4kcal, **Fats:** 27g, **Carbohydrates:** 28.5g, **Protein:** 9g

8. Broccoli Dal Curry

Ready in: 1 hr. 30 mins.

Serves: 4

Difficulty: easy

Ingredients:

- 2 onions (medium), chopped

- 4 tbsp. Of butter or 4 tbsp. of ghee

- 1 tsp. of chili powder

- 2 tsp. of cumin

- 1 1/2 tsp. of black pepper

- 1 tsp. of ground coriander

- 1 cup of red lentil

- 2 tsp. of turmeric

- juice of 1 lemon

- 2 broccoli (medium), chopped

- 3 cups of chicken broth

- ½ cup of dried coconut (optional)

- 1 tsp. of salt

- 1 tbsp. of flour

- 1 cup of coarsely chopped cashews (optional)

Directions:

- In a saucepan, melt the butter and brown the onions.

- Chili powder, cumin, pepper, coriander, and turmeric are all good additions.

- Do 1 minute of stirring and cooking

- Add the lentils, broth, lemon juice, and, if using, the coconut.

- Bring to a boil, then lower to low heat and cook for 55 minutes (if the batter is too thick, you might need to put in a little hot water).

- Do 7 minutes of steaming broccoli

- Set aside broccoli after submerging it in cold water.

- Remove 1/3 cup of the lentil mixture's liquid.

- To get a smooth paste, mix in the flour.

- Return to the pan and stir in the broccoli, salt, and nuts, if desired.

- Cook for 5 minutes on low heat.

- Over Basmati rice, serve.

Nutritional values per serving:

Total Calories: 445kcal, **Fats:** 138g, **Carbohydrates:** 59g, **Protein:** 25.7g

9. Sheet Pan Chicken & Brussels sprouts

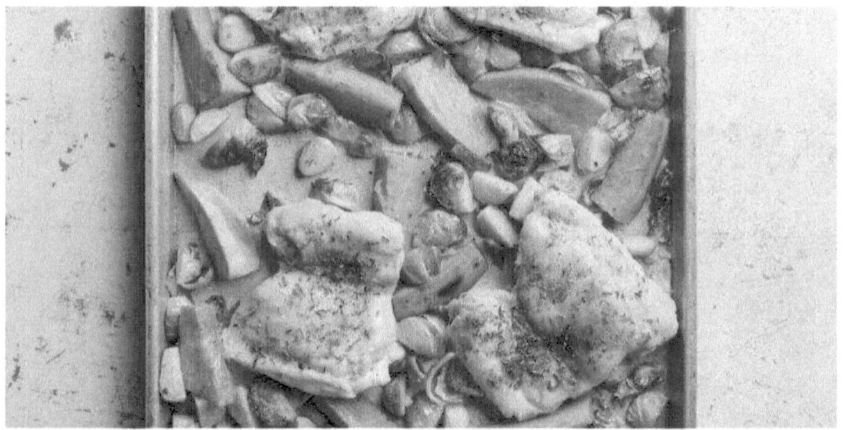

Ready in: 40 mins.

Serves: 4

Difficulty: easy

Ingredients:

- 1 and 1⁄2 cups of Brussels sprouts, halved

- 4 chicken thighs (skin on)

- 4 carrots, cut on the bias

- 1 tsp. of herbes de Provence

- 3 tbsp. of olive oil

Directions:

- Preheat the oven up to 400 degrees Fahrenheit.

- Toss sliced veggies with 1 and 1/2 tbsp. Olive oil, 1/2 tsp. Herbs, salt and black pepper in a bowl. Rub the veggies all over.

- Arrange the vegetables onto a sheet pan.

- In the same bowl, place the chicken thighs. Drizzle with 1and 1/2 tablespoons olive oil, and 1/2 tablespoons herbs, and season with salt and pepper. Rub the chicken all over.

- Place the chicken in the pan.

- Roast for 30-35 minutes, or till chicken is cooked through.

- Turn the oven towards broil & cook for 1-2 minutes if you desire a crispier chicken or vegetable skin. If you don't keep an eye on it, it will burn.

Nutritional values per serving:

Total Calories: 323.4kcal, **Fats:** 222g, **Carbohydrates:** 7.9g, **Protein:** 17.6g

Dinner Recipes

1. No-Bean Chili

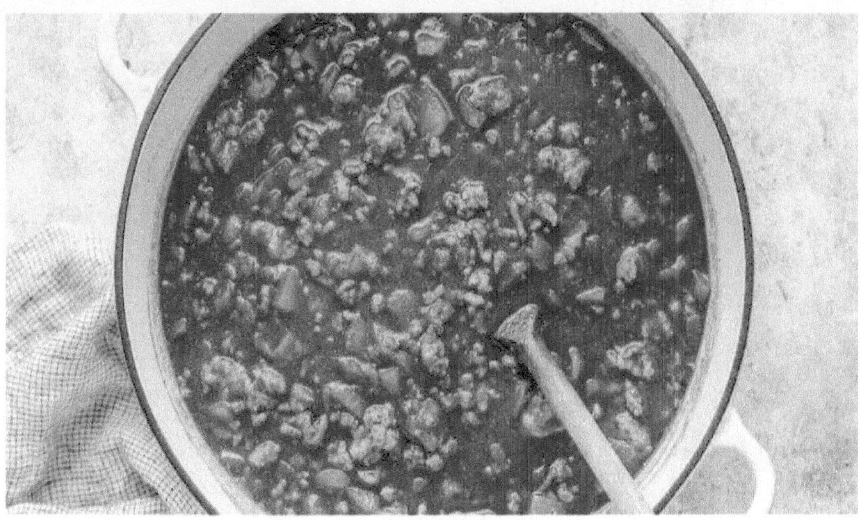

Ready in: 1 hr. 30 mins.

Serves: 4

Difficulty: medium

Ingredients:

- 4 minced garlic cloves

- 1 lb. of ground beef, grass-fed (or lamb)

- 1 finely diced onion

- 1 finely diced zucchini

- 1 cup of beef or chicken broth

- 2 tbsp. of tomato paste

- 1 tsp. of cayenne pepper

- 2 tsp. of chili powder

- 1 tsp. of cumin

- ½ tsp. of black pepper

- 1 tsp. of salt

- ½ tsp. of chili flakes

- 2 tbsp. of Bulletproof Grass-Fed Ghee

- 1-2 tbsp. of Bulletproof Collagelatin

For garnish:

- 1 tsp. of fresh herbs

- 1 cup of coconut yogurt

Directions:

- Preheat the frying pan to medium-high heat. Fry the chopped onion & minced garlic in 1 tbsp. Of Grass-Fed Ghee till golden brown.

- Cook until the ground beef (or lamb) is browned with another tablespoon of Ghee.

- Season with spices, salt, tomato paste, pepper, and broth. Stir everything together and cook for 30 mins to an hour. Add 1-2 teaspoons of Collagelatin to speed up the thickening process.

- Taste the mixture and, if required, add more chili powder or cayenne pepper.

- Pour into a bowl, top with chives and chili flakes, and serve with coconut yogurt.

Nutritional values per serving:

Total Calories: 434kcal, **Fats:** 32g, **Carbohydrates:** 13g, **Protein:** 23g

2. Fish Cakes with Lemon Avocado Dipping Sauce

Ready in: 15 mins.

Serves: 6

Difficulty: easy

Ingredients:

- 1/4 cup of cilantro (leaves & stems)

- 1 pound of white boneless fish, raw (preferably local & wild-caught)

- Pinch of salt

- 1-2 cloves of garlic (optional)

- Pinch of some chili flakes

- Neutral oil for making your hands greasy, like avocado oil

- 1-2 tbsp. of grass-fed ghee or coconut oil for frying

For Dipping Sauce:

- 1 juiced lemon

- 2 avocados, ripe

- 2 tbsp. of water

- Pinch of salt

Directions:

- Combine the fish, garlic (if using), herbs, salt, chile, and fish in a food processor. Blitz till everything is evenly blended.

- Add ghee or coconut oil to a wide frying pan over medium-high heat and stir to coat.

- Roll the mixture of fish into 6 patties using oiled hands.

- Place the cakes in the hot frying pan. Cook till golden brown & cooked thoroughly on both sides.

- While the fish cakes are frying, combine all of the dipping sauce ingredients in a blender or small food processor (beginning with the lemon juice) and blitz till smooth and creamy. If desired, add extra salt or lemon juice to the mixture.

- When the fish cakes are done, reheat them up and serve with a dipping sauce.

Nutritional values per serving:

Total Calories: 69kcal, **Fats:** 6.5g, **Carbohydrates:** 6g, **Protein:** 1.1g

3. Baked Paleo Meatballs

Ready in: 30 mins.

Serves: 3

Difficulty: easy

Ingredients:

- 2 tbsp. of Grass-Fed Ghee

- 1 and 1/4 pounds of pastured ground beef

- 1 tbsp. of apple cider vinegar

- 1 tsp. of salt

- 1/2 tsp. of pepper

- 1/2 yellow onion (medium), minced

- 1/4 cup of rosemary (fresh), roughly chopped

- 2 cloves of garlic, minced

- Optional: 1 tsp. of red pepper flakes (crushed)

Directions:

- Preheat the oven up to 350 degrees Fahrenheit.

- Put all of the meatball ingredients in a mixing bowl and mix everything together with your hands until everything is thoroughly incorporated.

- Roll the batter into small balls on a baking pan lined with parchment paper, using a little over a spoonful of ingredients per meatball.

- Bake for 20 minutes, or until cooked through. After all, meatballs have been rolled and put on paper.

- Allow cooling before serving, then store in the airtight container in the freezer or fridge.

Nutritional values per serving:

Total Calories: 474kcal, **Fats:** 21.7g, **Carbohydrates:** 5.6g, **Protein:** 61.3g

---

4. Grilled Lemon Salmon

Ready in: 27 mins.

Serves: 4

Difficulty: easy

Ingredients:

- ½ tsp. of pepper

- 2 tsp. of fresh dill

- ½ tsp. of salt

- 1 1/2 lbs. of salmon fillets

- 1/2 tsp. of garlic powder

- 1/4 cup of packed brown sugar

- 3 tbsp. of water

- 1 cube of chicken bouillon

- 3 tbsp. of oil

- 4 tbsp. of green onions, finely chopped

- 3 tbsp. of soy sauce

- 2 slices of onions, separated into rings

- 1 thinly sliced lemon

Directions:

- Season the salmon with dill, pepper, salt, and garlic powder.

- Fill a small glass pan halfway with water.

- Combine the sugar, chicken broth, soy sauce, oil, and green onions in a mixing bowl.

- Pour the sauce over the fish.

- Cover & chill for 1 hour, turning halfway through.

- Drain and toss out the marinade.

- Place lemon & onion on top of the grill over medium heat.

- Cook for 10-15 minutes or until the fish is cooked through.

Nutritional values per serving:

Total Calories: 380.7kcal, **Fats:** 161g, **Carbohydrates:** 17.3g, **Protein:** 37g

5. Club Tilapia Parmesan

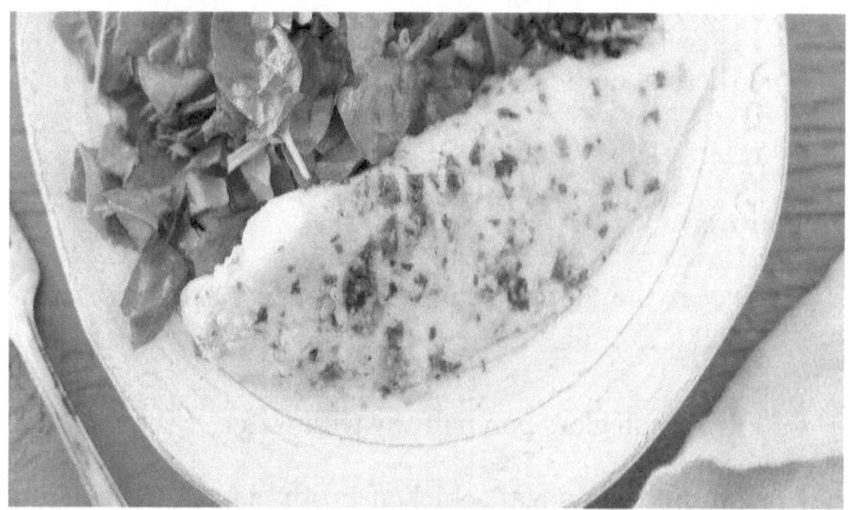

Ready in: 35 mins.

Serves: 4

Difficulty: easy

Ingredients:

- 2 tbsp. of lemon juice

- 2 lbs. of tilapia fillets

- 1⁄2 cup of grated parmesan cheese

- 3 tbsp. of mayonnaise

- 4 tbsp. of butter, room temperature

- 3 tbsp. of green onions, finely chopped

- 1⁄4 tsp. of dried basil

- 1⁄4 tsp. of seasoning salt

- 1 dash of hot pepper sauce

- Some black pepper

Directions:

- Preheat the oven up to 350 degrees Fahrenheit.

- Arrange the fillets in a single layer in a greased jelly roll or baking dish pan (13-by-9-inch).

- Fillets should not be stacked.

- Apply some juice to the top.

- Combine the cheese, mayonnaise, butter, onions, and spices in a mixing bowl.

- With a fork, thoroughly combine the ingredients.

- Bake the fish for 20 minutes in a preheated oven or until it begins to flake.

- Spread the cheese mixture on top and bake for 5 minutes or until golden brown.

- The length of time it takes to bake the fish will be determined by its thickness.

- Keep an eye on the fish to make sure it doesn't overcook.

Note: This fish may also be cooked in the broiler.

- Let 3–4 minutes in the broiler or until nearly done.

- Broil for another 2 - 3 minutes, or until cheese is browned.

Nutritional values per serving:

Total Calories: 376.8kcal, **Fats:** 170g, **Carbohydrates:** 1.4g, **Protein:** 50.6g

---

6. Baked Mahi Mahi

Ready in: 40 mins.

Serves: 4

Difficulty: easy

Ingredients:

- 1 juiced lemon

- 2 lbs. of Mahi Mahi (four fillets)

- 1/4 tsp. of garlic salt

- 1 cup of mayonnaise

- 1⁄4 tsp. of ground black pepper

- Some breadcrumbs

- 1⁄4 cup of finely chopped white onion

Directions:

- Preheat the oven up to 425 degrees Fahrenheit.

- Place the fish on a baking dish after rinsing it. Squeeze lemon juice over the fish, then season with salt and pepper.

- Spread mayonnaise & chopped onions on the fish. Bake for 25 minutes at 425°F with breadcrumbs on top.

Nutritional values per serving:

Total Calories: 201.9kcal, **Fats:** 14g, **Carbohydrates:** 2.5g, **Protein:** 42.2g

7. Sweet Potato & Black Bean Burrito

Ready in: 1 hr. 5 mins.

Serves: 8-12

Difficulty: easy

Ingredients:

- 1⁄2 tsp. of salt

- 5 cups of cubed peeled sweet potatoes

- 2 tsp. of broth or other vegetable oil

- 4 cloves of garlic, minced (or pressed)

- 3 ½ cups of diced onions

- 1 tbsp. of minced green chili pepper, fresh

- 4 tsp. of ground coriander

- 4 tsp. of ground cumin

- 4 and ½ cups of black beans, cooked (three cans (15-ounce), drained)

- 2 tbsp. of fresh lemon juice

- 2/3 cup of cilantro leaf, lightly packed

- 1 tsp. of salt

- Fresh salsa

- 12 flour tortillas (10 inches)

Directions:

- Preheat the oven up to 350 degrees Fahrenheit.

- In a medium saucepan, combine the sweet potatoes, salt, and enough water to cover them.

- Cover & bring to boil, then reduce to low heat and cook until the vegetables are soft, approximately 10 minutes.

- Drain the water and put it aside.

- Warm the oil into a medium saucepan or skillet and add the garlic, onions, and chile while the sweet potatoes are frying.

- Cover and simmer over medium-low heat, stirring periodically, for approximately 7 minutes, or until the onions are soft.

- Cook, stirring regularly, for another 2 to 3 minutes after adding the cumin and coriander.

- Take the pan off the heat and put it aside.

- Puree the cilantro, black beans, salt, lemon juice, and cooked sweet potatoes in a food processor till smooth (or you can mash the ingredients into a big bowl by hand).

- Add the sautéed onions and spices to the mixture of sweet potatoes in a large mixing bowl.

- A big baking dish should be lightly oiled.

- Fill each tortilla with approximately 2/3 - 3/4 cup of the filling, wrap it up, and lay it seam-side down in the baking dish.

- Bake for 30 minutes, or until boiling hot, covered securely with foil.

- Serve with salsa on top.

Nutritional values per serving:

Total Calories: 575.2kcal, **Fats:** 92g, **Carbohydrates:** 102g, **Protein:** 19.8g

---

8. Sweet Potato Curry with Chickpeas and Spinach

Ready in: 30 mins.

Serves: 6

Difficulty: easy

Ingredients:

- 1 -2 tsp. of canola oil

- ½ sweet onions (large), chopped or two scallions, thinly sliced

- 2 tbsp. of curry powder

- 1 tsp. of cinnamon

- 1 tbsp. of cumin

- 10 ounces of spinach (fresh), stemmed, washed & coarsely chopped

- 1 can of chickpeas (14 1/2 ounce), rinsed & drained

- 2 sweet potatoes (large), peeled & diced (about 2 lbs.)

- ½ cup of water

- 1/4 cup of chopped cilantro (fresh) for garnish

- 1 can of diced tomatoes (14 1/2 ounce), can use fresh if available

- brown rice or basmati rice for serving

Directions:

- Heat 1-2 tsp. Vegetable or canola oil over medium heat while sweet potatoes are cooking.

- Add the onions and cook for 2-3 minutes, or till they soften.

- Stir in the cumin, curry powder, and cinnamon to uniformly cover the onions with spices.

- Stir in the tomatoes and their juices, as well as the chickpeas.

- Increase the heat to a hard simmer for approximately 1 min or 2 after adding 1/2 cup of water.

- Then, a few fistfuls at a time, add some fresh spinach, stirring to cover with the cooking liquid.

- When all of the spinach has been put into the pan, cover & cook for 3 minutes, or until barely wilted.

- Stir cooked sweet potatoes into the liquid to coat them.

- Cook for another 3 to 5 minutes, or till all the flavors are fully blended.

- Serve immediately after transferring to a serving dish and tossing with fresh cilantro.

- This meal goes well with brown or basmati rice.

Nutritional values per serving:

Total Calories: 166.5kcal, **Fats:** 21g, **Carbohydrates:** 32g, **Protein:** 6.8g

9. Cajun Potato, Shrimp/ Prawn & Avocado Salad

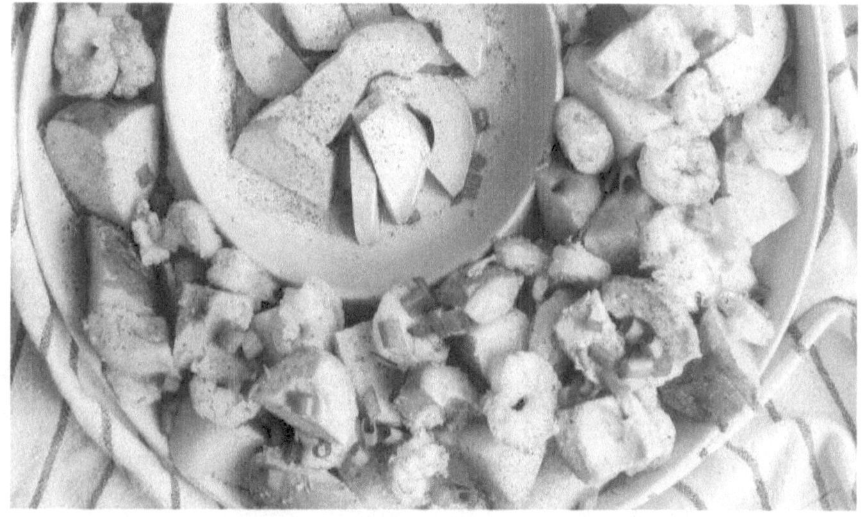

Ready in: 30 mins.

Serves: 2

Difficulty: easy

Ingredients:

- 1 tbsp. of olive oil

- 300g of potatoes

- 250 g of king prawns (cooked & peeled, 8 oz.)

- 2 finely sliced spring onions

- 1 clove of garlic (minced)

- 2 tsp. of Cajun seasoning

- 1 cup of alfalfa sprout

- 1 peeled avocado (stoned & diced)

- Some salt

Directions:

- Cook the potatoes for 10 to 15 minutes, or until cooked, in a big saucepan of slightly salted boiling water. Drain thoroughly.

- In a wok or big nonstick frying pan/skillet, heat the oil.

- Stir in the prawns, spring onions, garlic, and Cajun spice till the prawns are heated, about 2 to 3 minutes.

- Cook for another minute after adding the potatoes.

- Transfer to serving plates and garnish with avocado & alfalfa sprouts before serving.

Nutritional values per serving:

Total Calories: 435.6kcal, **Fats:** 207g, **Carbohydrates:** 37.9g, **Protein:** 23.1g

Three-Course Meal Plan for 1 Week

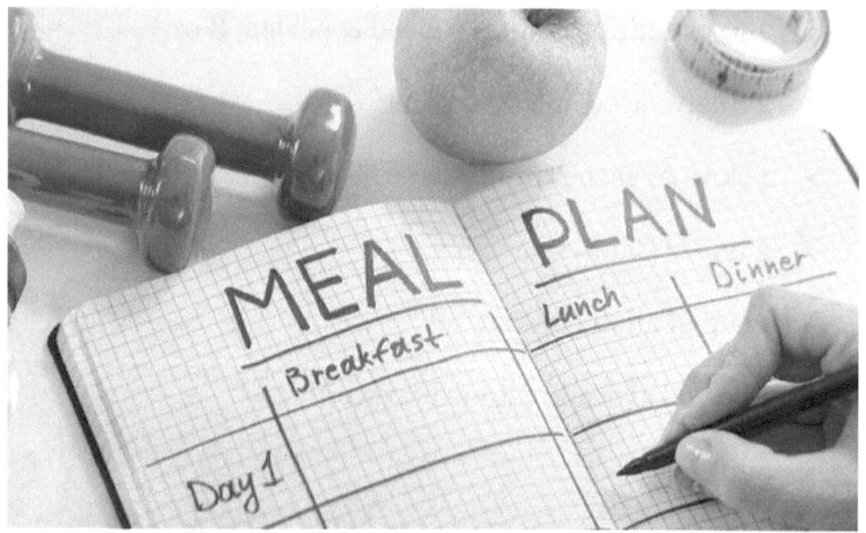

From previously mentioned recipes

Day 1:

Breakfast: 1. Buddha Breakfast Bowl

Lunch: 1. Avocado Quesadillas

Dinner: 1. No-Bean Chili

Day 2:

Breakfast: 2. Garlic Spinach and Smoked Salmon Breakfast Sandwich

Lunch: 2. Cheesy Veggie Packed Chicken Salad

Dinner: 3. Baked Paleo Meatballs

Day 3:

Breakfast: 4. Breakfast Pizza

Lunch: 4. Chicken Breasts & Avocado Tapenade

Dinner: 4. Grilled Lemon Salmon

Day 4:

Breakfast: 6. Coconut Flour Breakfast Pancakes

Lunch: 5. Lamb Tacos & Cauliflower Tortillas

Dinner: 6. Baked Mahi Mahi

Day 5:

Breakfast: 7. Perfect Basic Hard Boiled Eggs

Lunch: 6. Thai Grilled Steak with Low-Carb Salad

Dinner: 7. Sweet Potato & Black Bean Burrito

Day 6:

Breakfast: 8. Peach Smoothie

Lunch: 9. Broccoli Dal Curry

Dinner: 8. Sweet Potato Curry with Chickpeas and Spinach

Day 7:

Breakfast: 9. Avocado & Poached Eggs Toast

Lunch: 10. Sheet Pan Chicken & Brussels sprouts

Dinner: 3. Baked Paleo Meatballs

Conclusion

It is a luxury to grow older. "If I had known I would be going to survive this long, I might well have taken good care of my body," many individuals have said. For many individuals, there is undoubtedly much truth in that remark. While you can't change what you've done or didn't do years previously, you can go on and do your best to look after yourself today. Regular exercise & a good diet seem to be essential for practically every element of your evolving physique. So, keep moving, eat properly, and enjoy the remainder of your day. While aging is not a sickness in and of itself, it is a health risk for several ailments. This does not imply you will get an age-related illness; rather, as you become older, you are more prone to develop certain disorders. Physiological mechanisms like inflammation, exposure to radiation (such as UV radiation from the sun) & pollutants, the impact of lifestyle variables such as smoking, food, & fitness levels, and also normal wear and tear may all hasten the pace of decline in various persons.

Many research initiatives are undertaken throughout the globe to understand the impact of aging on the human body and to establish which problems are unavoidable as you age and which may be avoided. Most women accumulate belly fat beyond the age of 50. Diabetes, dementia, heart disease, and some malignancies have all been related to belly fat. If you're in your 40s and have one of these illnesses, follow your doctor's eating recommendations. Women lose muscle mass twice as quickly as males after 50. Your core muscles that support your abdomen lose the most weight. Muscle loss is also caused by crash diets (eating an extremely low-calorie diet in order to lose weight quickly and in a short period of time) and not utilizing your muscles. Although most women gain more weight as they get older, this isn't always the case. Step up your exercise level and eat a balanced diet to avoid menopausal weight gain.

Intermittent fasting (IF), for example, has been shown to be an effective way to maintain and enhance a healthy lifestyle. Fasting may be done for a variety of reasons, including weight loss, detoxification, and religious reasons. There's been a significant quantity of scientific study that supports the health advantages of fasting. Despite the fact that it has mostly been tested on animals, the findings are nonetheless encouraging. Fasting lowers oxidative stress, improves memory, retains learning, and improves disease biomarkers. Remember that weight reduction at any age needs long-term adjustments in food and activity habits. Make a commitment to a healthy lifestyle and get the benefits.

Glossary

1. **Affirmations:** Positive phrases that may help you fight and overcome self-sabotaging & negative beliefs.

2. **Alzheimer's disease:** It is a chronic illness that starts with modest memory loss and progresses to the loss of capacity to converse and react to the surroundings.

3. **Anorexia nervosa:** It is a kind of eating disorder marked by an extremely low weight and a strong fear of weight gain.

4. **Appetite:** a strong desire to consume food, generally as a result of hunger.

5. **Arthritis:** Swelling and discomfort of 1 or more joints.

6. **Autophagy:** Hunger and certain disorders cause the body to consume its own tissue like a metabolic mechanism.

7. **BMI:** The Body mass index is a measurement of body fat for adult men & women based on weight and height.

8. **Bone density:** The quantity of bone minerals inside the bone tissue is measured by bone density, also known as bone mineral density.

9. **Bulimia:** It is a psychiatric eating disorder characterized by binge eating episodes (consuming a big quantity of food in 1 sitting).

10. **Calorie deficit:** It happens when a person's daily calorie intake is lower than their daily calorie expenditure.

11. **Circadian rhythms:** These are 24-hour cycles of physical, mental, and behavioral changes.

12. **Constipation:** It is a state in which a person's bowel motions are painful or infrequent.

13. **Dementia:** It is defined as a loss of cognitive function, remembering, thinking, and reasoning to the point that it affects a person's everyday life and activities.

14. **Detoxification:** The liver is primarily responsible for detoxification, which is the physiological or therapeutic elimination of poisonous chemicals from living organisms, such as the human body.**Endurance exercises:** Walking, running, swimming, riding, and jumping rope are considered endurance exercises that raise your breathing & heart rate.

15. **Epilepsy:** It is a neurological illness wherein brain activity gets aberrant, resulting in seizures or

episodes of odd behavior, feelings, and even loss of consciousness.

16. **Ghrelin:** It is a hormone generated by enteroendocrine cells in the gastrointestinal system, particularly the stomach that enhances the desire to eat.

17. **Glycemic control:** It refers to a person with diabetes Mellitus's ability to maintain normal blood sugar (glucose) levels.

18. **HGH:** Human growth hormone (HGH) is the secret to reducing the ageing process. Growth hormone supports early development and aids in the maintenance of tissues & organs throughout life. It is created by the pituitary gland, a little organ at the center of the skull.

19. **Hysterectomies:** the condition in which the uterus is surgically removed.

20. **Insulin resistance:** It is a disorder in which cells in the muscles, fat, & liver do not react effectively to insulin and are unable to utilize glucose from the blood as an energy source.

21. **Insulin sensitivity:** It is the degree to which the body's cells respond to insulin.

22. **Irritability:** It is a state of agitation that occurs

when you are frustrated or irritated.

23. **Ketones:** When your cells don't receive enough glucose (blood sugar), your body produces ketones.

24. **Menopause:** It is defined as the total cessation of menstrual periods.

25. **Metabolic shift:** Body's preference for fatty acids & fatty acid-derived ketones over glucose consumption via glycogenolysis.

26. **Metabolism:** The process through which your body transforms what you eat & drink into energy.

27. **MMC:** Migrating Motor Complex is cyclic, repeating motility pattern in the stomach & small intestine that occurs while fasting and is halted by eating.

28. **Nausea:** a strong desire to vomit.

29. **Osteoporosis:** It is a disease that causes bones to become increasingly weak and prone to breaking.

30. **Oxidative stress:** It is a condition in which the body's free radicals & antioxidants are out of equilibrium, causing cell & tissue damage. Oxidative stress is a normal occurrence that contributes to the aging process.

31. **Parkinson's disease:** It is a movement illness that produces unintentional or involuntary movements such as stiffness, shaking, and balance and

coordination problems.

32.   **Sedentary:** in contrast to an active lifestyle, a sedentary lifestyle involves little or no physical activity & exercise.

33.   **Sleep apnea:** It is a potentially fatal sleep disease in which breathing stops and begins frequently.

34.   **TRF (time-restricted feeding):** In time-restricted feeding, individuals consume their regular food but only for a certain amount of time each day.